First Aid in the Workplace

Lord Taylor and his colleagues are pioneers in a new approach to the teaching of first aid in industry. Starting out by studying what first aiders actually *do* in factories and other workplaces, they concentrate on the practical and detailed care of the accidents and illnesses that commonly occur.

In this edition special attention is devoted to injuries of the hands, feet and eyes, wound cleaning and protection from oil and solvents. Modern methods of dealing with shock, fractures, gassing and chemical splashes are fully considered. The care of the unconscious patient and simple methods of transport of the injured are clearly explained and illustrated. In addition a special precautionary note has been included concerning AIDS and hepatitis B. The duties of the first aider and the statutory contents of industrial first aid boxes are covered in detail, reflecting the most recent first aid legislation and practice, and a separate chapter on training underlines the need for qualified first aiders in every area of industry and commerce

This book was first published in 1960 under the title *First Aid in the Factory*. Readers will have noted the change in the title for the sixth edition. The simple fact is that the number of factories in Britain is declining and that of other workplaces is correspondingly rising. The law requires first aid facilities in both.

We hope that this book will prove as effective in meeting the needs of new readers in new situations as it has in factories in the past. It meets fully the requirements of those who learn, teach and practise first aid at work.

Courses based on the teaching given in this book are recognised by the Health and Safety Executive. Individual firms or groups of firms with their own doctor or suitably qualified nursing officer, can either apply to the Health and Safety Executive for approval of a course of their own choice, or they can affiliate to the Harlow Industrial Health Service for first aid training, for help and advice in the planning of courses and the examination of candidates.

Those who are already running their own approved courses will find *First Aid in the Workplace* an invaluable teaching aid and reference book for their students.

First Aid in the Workplace

Sixth edition

Lord Taylor of Harlow
B Sc, M D, Hon L L D, FRCP, FRCGP, FRCPsych, FFOM

and

Dr Patricia Elliott
MD, MFOM, DPH, DIH, DMS

With the assistance of

Prudence D Wright
SRN, OHNC

Foreword by

Rt Hon Lord Robens
PC

Pitman

Pitman Publishing
128 Long Acre, London WC2E 9AN

First published in Great Britain as *First Aid in the Factory* 1960
Second edition 1962
Third edition 1967
Fourth edition 1973
Fifth edition 1981
Sixth edition 1988

© Lord Taylor 1967

British Library Cataloguing in Publication Data

Taylor, Stephen James Lake Taylor, *Baron*
    First aid in the workplace. — 6th ed.
    1. First aid in illness and injury
    I. Title II. Elliott, Patricia
    III. Wright, Prudence D. IV. Taylor,
    Stephen James Lake Taylor, *Baron*. First
    aid in the factory
    616.02'52

ISBN 0–273–02858–8

Produced by Longman Singapore Publishers (Pte) Ltd.
Printed in Singapore

Contents

Illustrations

x Illustrations

Foreword

An occurrence which in any way diminishes Britain's economic progress is necessarily a bad thing. When it is accompanied by injury, it is doubly bad because of the pain and suffering which ensues. What must be surprising to most people is to learn that the number of days lost in any year is greater, as a result of injury at the workplace, than by the much more publicised industrial disputes. The public eye has not in fact been focused on injuries at work and it has been left to comparatively few individuals and associations to awaken the public consciousness.

My own experience on the subject was in the early 1930s when, as a trade union representative, and later as a full-time trade union official, I was responsible for making claims for compensation. In 1960 I became Chairman of the National Coal Board, now British Coal, perhaps the most accident prone industry in the country by the very nature and conditions of work.

At a later stage I was invited by the Government to chair a working party to enquire into the health and safety of people at work and make recommendations. The evidence was a revelation. The recommendations, which led to the appointment of the Health and Safety Executive, were approved by Parliament and have been highly successful.

By that time, however, I was involved in the details and resultant problems suffered by those injured at their place of work. But whilst I was still studying the problem, Lord Taylor and his colleagues were acting. In 1960 the first edition of this book, then called *First Aid in the Factory* came off the press. Lord Taylor and his colleagues at the Harlow Industrial Health Service had done an excellent job. Their main emphasis lay upon the need for a sufficient number of well-trained first aiders, at least one to each first aid box that the law required.

There is still a lack of adequately trained first aiders, and as they are, as Lord Taylor describes, at the front line of defence against occupational ill-health, it is absolutely essential that management should provide proper facilities and encouragement to ensure that there are sufficient expertly trained first aiders on the payroll to cope with the forty million industrial injuries which all require immediate treatment that occur each year. The quality of first aiders is crucial and they need a first class manual.

Lord Taylor and his colleagues have produced this book which the first aiders will value and enjoy. They will find it highly informative, and it will enable them to deal with injuries effectively and efficiently at first hand. No first aider should be without it and modern forward-looking management should ensure they have it. It is certainly, without question, one of the very best first aid manuals available.

Alfred Robens
PC, Hon LLD
(The Rt Hon Lord Robens of Woldingham)

Lord Stephen Taylor died in February 1988 whilst the Sixth Edition was being prepared for publication.

Acknowledgments and thanks

In this new edition I have been joined by Dr Patricia Elliott as co-author as I am no longer actively engaged in first aid teaching. We must first offer special thanks to the Rt Hon Lord Robens of Woldingham for agreeing to write a foreword. The monumental report of his Committee on Health and Safety at work has changed the whole pattern of occupational medicine, and with it, occupational first-aid. Special thanks are also due to Dr Austin Eagger, the founding father of the group Industrial Health Services in Britain. His foreword has graced our pages for 27 years and five editions. Like me he has long since retired from active industrial practice, and he has kindly agreed to step down to make way for Lord Robens. Thus, one pioneer is succeeded by another.

In preparing this and previous editions of the book I have been helped by the following people and organisations, in particular, the staff and Council of the Harlow Industrial Health Service, notably Mrs Prudence Wright SRN, OHNC and Mrs Evelyn Craven SRN, and more recently Dr Celia Palmer, Mrs Molly Hitchcock and Mrs Anne Thorpe SRN, OHNC. Many former staff members contributed to earlier editions, among them Drs Barbara Ely, B S Laing, O Ross, the late Dr W N Booth, Mr Geoffrey Fisk FRCS and the late Dr Leo Bourne, and, members of the lay staff, Mrs Joan Lloyd, Mrs Jay Ellis and Mrs Barbara Dunce.

My thanks are also due to the staff of the Health and Safety Executive, on whose experience we have frequently drawn.

Many individuals have given help and expert advice, notably Prof. Richard Schilling, Dr David Gullick, Dr Robert Piper, Dr J P W Hughes, Dr R H Green, Dr R Mellanby, Dr J R Busvine, Mr J D Peacock, the late Lord Platt, the late Mr Ruscoe Clarke and Dr C H Hoskyn.

The line drawings are the work of Miss Sheila Dunn.

Finally I must thank the Nuffield Provincial Hospitals Trust, whose initial stimulation and generosity made possible the creation of the Harlow Industrial Health Service, and most important, the industrialists and workers of Harlow, in particular the first aiders whose work has shown that health in industry is a proper object for the united efforts of management and labour.

Lord Taylor of Harlow
November 1987

1 A new look at first aid

Introduction

For many years, first aid was the Cinderella of the health services, a poor
relation of nursing and minor surgery. While the science of medicine was
advancing at break-neck speed, first aid stood still, drably dressed in
garments long out of fashion. But at last things are changing. In the
twenty seven years since this book first appeared much thought and care
has been given to bring first aid practice and teaching up to date, so it
may be said that Cinderella is going to her first modern dancing class!

There is no reason why first aid should be dull and dowdy. Approached
in the spirit of scientific inquiry, it presents a fascinating series of
problems for both learner and teacher. It is an exercise in social behaviour, applied medicine and surgery, and teaching method. The account
given here of first aid at work is not in any sense final. First aid must
advance with the advance of medicine itself; and we feel sure that, even
in the light of existing experience, what we have to say can be bettered in
many ways. But if we only unlock the straitjacket of the past, we shall
have done our job.

It all started by chance. When we set out in 1955 to create a group
industrial health service, we found we needed first aiders. We found that
we had to supply and stock first aid boxes in small factories. We were
shocked at some of the things the law compelled us to put in these boxes,
so, as a first step, we began by finding out what first aiders in industry
really have to *do*. We started with a work study or job analysis and soon
found that at that time teaching bore little relation to the occupational
first aider's actual needs. So we had to work out a new scheme of
teaching, directly related to the situations which face the first aider in the
factory, shop or office, on the building site or the farm. This book is a
result of that scheme.

In every factory or workplace, first aiders have a real part to play. But
the emphasis of their work is different from, for example, first aid on the
roads. Conventional first aid courses devote much space to the control of

serious haemorrhage, fractures of the long bones and other forms of severe injury. Happily, in industry, serious accidents are comparatively rare; when they do occur, the first aider must know what to do and how far to go. But expert help is usually so quickly available that heroic first aid is seldom needed.

The day-to-day picture of first aid at work is rather a stream of minor injuries and minor ailments, small cuts and burns, colds and headaches. Many of these the first aider will have to treat alone and they will never be seen by a trained nurse or a doctor. In so doing, the first aider is stepping beyond conventional first aid and is, in fact, giving full treatment. At first sight this may seem wrong to the doctor or to the trained nurse. But pause and think for a moment. In the home we treat small cuts and headaches ourselves; if we did not do so, the health services would break down under the strain. There are far too many very small companies for nurses and doctors to treat minor injuries and ailments in each and this is where first aiders come into their own.

In undertaking full treatment of minor injuries and ailments, the first aider is shouldering a serious responsibility and must know exactly what the job is, its limits, and when to call for help. Given this knowledge and given the tools for the job, the first aider is the real first line of defence in the health care of people at work. In our experience, all too often first aiders have neither the knowledge nor the tools. Here we set out to describe the tools they ought to have, and the basic essentials they must know.

The first aider at work – responsibilities

The experiences of a first aider at work differ from those of someone undertaking conventional first aid in the following ways:

1 The number of patients the first aider can expect to treat is much greater. First aiders in the home or on the road may not even have to use their skills once a month, but a first aider at work may deal with five, ten or twenty people in the course of a day.
2 The nature of the work is different – there may be special risks and dangers to be dealt with in special ways, and, above all, there is likely to be a stream of minor injuries to be coped with. A first aider at work, then, has to become a specialist in the proper treatment of such injuries.
3 Dressings and other materials are, or always should be, at hand. There is therefore little need for improvisation.
4 In larger organisations skilled nursing or medical help is often

immediately available or readily called if necessary. Except in the more remote places a hospital can be reached fairly quickly and so the first aider need not be alone for long. Faced with serious injury the first aider need only know what to do until help arrives.

The first aider at work – limits of responsibility

The first aider must *never* be treated as an alternative to an occupational health nurse – this would be damaging both for patients and for first aiders themselves. A good first aider is skilled in the job but the limits of first aid responsibility *must* be clearly defined. First aiders, then:

- *must not* attempt to become semi-skilled doctors or nurses;
- *are not* ambulance workers – ambulance workers are trained and skilled in the transport of the severely injured whereas most first aiders have little or no experience in this area.
- *must* think for themselves but *must not* attempt to make precise diagnoses of all major conditions. They are not competent for this – the first task is simply to decide quickly whether the illness or injury is or is not within the scope of first aid treatment.
- *must* be able to give initial life-saving treatment to serious injuries.
- *must* know where and how to refer the patient for further treatment and know how to use the emergency services.

In this book we shall introduce all the most common complaints which first aiders are likely to encounter. If they have a sound practical knowledge of how to deal with common complaints well, first aiders will be better prepared to cope in an emergency.

The first aider in the occupational health team

The first aider is on the front line in the battle for health but cannot do the job well without proper support. This means every first aider ought to be part of an organised industrial health service. Such a service already exists to a greater or lesser degree in many large firms. Trained nurses are usually on duty throughout the main working periods, with doctors available or on call. In medium-sized or smaller organizations, however, this is still rare. Only about one per cent of all workplaces employing fewer than 250 people, for example, have any proper medical services. Smaller companies cannot afford the overheads involved, as the volume of work would not justify a full-time nurse. One answer is that organizations in the same area pool their resources to a local industrial health service.

The Nuffield Provincial Hospitals Trust originally sponsored three such health services – on the Slough Trading Estate, at Harlow New Town and in the Central Middlesex area. Group industrial health services have also been established at Dundee, Rochdale, West Bromwich, Milton Keynes, Telford and Newcastle.

These services can bring to the workers in smaller organizations the same level of industrial medical care as is enjoyed by workers in the very largest firms. Each member company contributes financially according to the number of employees, so that a firm with perhaps only 20 workers can always have available a service which is paid for on behalf of 4,000 or more workers.

Practising first aid within the occupational health team

As we can see from Table 1.1, no matter how large or small the organization the first aider is a valuable member of the healthcare team.

In any substantial occupational health service, whether serving one or many workplaces, doctors and nurses must be fully mobile. Yet it will never be possible for them to be everywhere when they are needed. This is why it is essential to have trained first aiders on the shopfloor and in the office – they will be the first to see almost every casualty. First aiders will themselves deal with a defined range of minor casualties so their judgment is the first vital link in the chain of efficient medical care. The most important single lesson to learn is *when to pass on a patient or call for help*. The doctor has to learn this, too, and the occupational nurse also. Every one of us has limitations and success in all medical work depends on our capacity to recognise them. The first aider working alone in a small organization should ideally have a doctor or group of doctors and nurses to call on when help is needed and must be ready to send on any patient needing more than first aid care.

We look forward to the day when all first aiders are associated with local or area occupational health services or have fully staffed medical departments within their companies.

The first aider and health and safety

Besides playing a part in treatment, the first aider has another function: to be an exponent of health and safety within the workplace. Nowadays

Table 1.1   The first aider within the health team.

	Staff available	Facilities	Outside medical help
Occupational health centre servicing several firms, e.g. Group Occupation Health Services	Medical director Doctors working regular sessions in the individual firm and in the centre Full-time nurses and part-time nurses working regular sessions in individual firms and in the centre First aiders	Fully equipped medical centre	Liaison with and referral to local hospital and emergency services
Large factories and offices	Full-time or part-time doctors Full-time nurses *or* Part-time nurses working regular sessions First aiders	Fully equipped medical treatment room First aid posts	Liaison with and referral to hospital and emergency services
Medium sized organizations	Possibly a part-time doctor/nurse First aiders	Ideally a medical room with first aid boxes and equipment First aid posts	Possibly a doctor on call Liaison with and referral to hospital and emergency services
Small organizations	First aiders	First aid boxes	Referral to hospital and emergency services.

it is almost a platitude to say that all workplaces should be healthy, safe and happy as well as vigorous and productive. Work ought to be enjoyed. Professional grumblers and carpers are producers of collective mental ill health. Nevertheless critical observation is constantly necessary. In the best regulated workplace, accidents will still happen. New machines and processes will always be coming along, with new risks and hazards to be overcome.

It is not our intention here to attempt to teach industrial safety or hygiene. The St John and Red Cross industrial first aid book has a helpful chapter on industrial safety. The Health and Safety Executive, the Royal Society for the Prevention of Accidents (RoSPA) and the British Safety Council all offer guidance for health and safety practitioners. There is also the excellent industrial health and safety exhibition centre of the Department of Employment which the first aider may visit. This is open from 10 a.m. to 5 p.m. from Monday to Friday and the address is:

97 Horseferry Road
London SW1

Learning and teaching

This book forms the basis for study for both those who learn and those who teach first aid. The needs of the one will not always be quite the same as those of the other; in particular, the theory behind a particular line of treatment may be essential knowledge for the teacher, yet may confuse the beginner. Training is dealt with in detail in Chapter 15 but before reading on note that besides knowledge, the good first aider must acquire certain qualities of behaviour. Indeed, a first aider can only apply knowledge effectively when these qualities have become a part of his or her approach to every patient. Good first aiders must be:

1 careful in their observations
2 accurate in their interrogation
3 honest in their judgment
4 ready to admit mistakes and learn from experience
5 clean, systematic and gentle in their treatment of patients
6 quiet, relaxed and unhurried in demeanour.

Re-read and ponder this list of qualities while working through each stage of this book!

Who should learn occupational first aid?

It is worth considering how many first aiders there should be in organizations of different sizes, and whether or not every worker in industry and commerce should receive some elementary teaching in first aid. Everyone should be conscious of the need for good 'house-keeping' and for the simple measures which can prevent accidents and promote safety in the workplace. Everyone should also be aware of the necessity for elementary hygiene if lavatories and canteens are to be as clean as they ought to be in the interests of health.

But not everyone can practise occupational first aid; if they attempted to do so, the result would be chaos. There must be one first aider responsible for each first aid box for each shift, one deputy ready to take over in case of absence or illness. It may be that these key first aiders will have had some general training before they learn occupational first aid as taught here. But our teaching can stand on its own, and the beginner who knows only what is written here will be able to cope well.

There is one final proviso. In some jobs there are special risks, for which special local instructions are needed. But the general principles and practice of first aid do not vary with locality. It is with the general picture of industrial and occupational first aid that we are now concerned.

2 The first aider's tools and tasks

The first aider at work starts with an advantage over first aiders elsewhere. British legislation lays down that tools for the job must be provided. Depending on the number of employees, the minimum and maximum contents of the first aid box are specified. Only when first aid services are supervised by a doctor or trained occupational health nurse may additional items be included. This chapter begins with a description of first aid boxes and the statutory contents and suggests other items it may be helpful to add. Figure 2.1 illustrates standard boxes and contents.

First aid boxes

First aid boxes and containers should be made of material suitable to protect the contents from damp and dust. Boxes must be clearly identified with a white cross on a green background, a provision necessary to conform with a European Common Market regulation.

In general any wooden boxes are superior to those made of metal or plastic. Some boxes supplied commercially have fronts which let down to provide a work space for the first aider. This is a good arrangement but unfortunately, the supporting chains are usually too flimsy.

Internally, every box should have enough room for any additional contents which may be recommended by trained medical help and a space in which bottles can be kept upright. This space must be *at least* 10 inches (25 cm) in height if it is to contain 20 oz (500 ml) bottles. We recommend spaces of:

Size of bottle	Dimensions
20 oz (500 ml)	10 × 6 × 4 inches (25 × 15 × 10 cm)
10 oz (250 ml)	8½ × 5 × 4 (25 × 13 × 10 cm)

Boxes supplied commercially seldom have enough space; consequently, in most small factories, dust-covered equipment decorates the top of the first aid box.

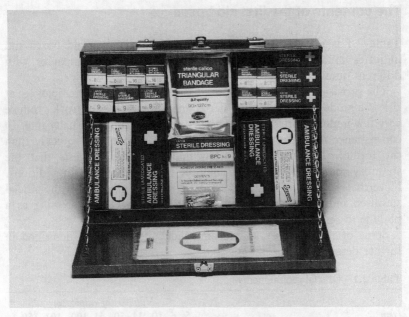

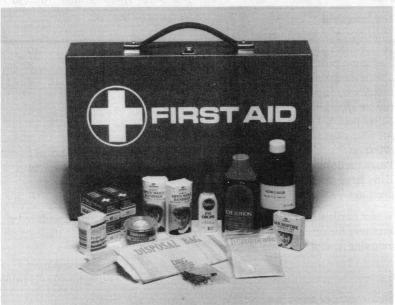

Figure 2.1 Standard first aid boxes. The official individual dressings are shown in the open box; additions recommended by the Harlow Industrial Health Service are shown in front of the closed box

The contents of the first aid boxes

Table 2.1 is a checklist of the official contents of first aid boxes and indicates minimum and maximum requirements for companies with different numbers of employees.

The provision of dressings on the basis of the number of employees at risk is a guide to the minimum needs only. Some types of work produce very few minor injuries; other types have a heavy minor casualty rate. In consequence the latter will use up first aid supplies more quickly than the former. Experience at Harlow and elsewhere suggests that the statutory contents of the boxes could be improved by certain additions. Nevertheless, most of the basic items are sound. In particular the official sterilised individual dressing is still the best emergency dressing as a prelude to removal for treatment elsewhere.

Some of the statutory and recommended items will be described in further detail.

Table 2.1   Official requirements

| Item | Numbers of employees | | | | |
	1–5	6–10	11–50	51–100	101–150
Guidance card	1	1	1	1	1
Individually wrapped sterile adhesive dressings	10	20	40	40	40
Sterile eye pads, with attachment	1	2	4	6	8
Triangular bandages	1	2	4	6	8
Sterile coverings for serious wounds (where applicable)	1	2	4	6	8
Safety pins	6	6	12	12	12
Medium sized sterile unmedicated dressings	3	6	8	10	12
Large sterile unmedicated dressings	1	2	4	6	10
Extra large sterile unmedicated dressings	1	2	4	6	8

Where sterile water or sterile normal saline in disposable containers needs to be kept near the first aid box because tap water is not available, at least the following quantities should be kept:

| | Number of employees | | | |
	1–10	11–50	51–100	101–150
Sterile water or saline in disposable containers (where tap water is not available)	1	3	6	6

In addition, protective clothing, e.g. disposable gloves, must be provided to protect the first aider when necessary.

Sterilised individual dressing (statutory requirement)

Standard sterilised individual dressing (*see* Fig. 2.2) is made in several sizes. In common use are:

---

medium (nos 8 and 9) for injured hands or feet; and
large (ambulance dressing no. 3) for other injured parts.

The dressing consists of a thick absorbent pad, with a layer of lint, or preferably gauze, on the side to be applied to the wound, and a roller bandage stitched to the other side. The whole forms a small roll, which is wrapped in paper and enclosed in a cardboard box. The dressing itself, inside the paper, is sterilised. Sometimes the pad may be medicated, but this is both unnecessary and undesirable. The bandage is rolled in such a way that when the paper covering has been torn off, the pad can be applied to a wound without being touched by the hand, and so remains germ-free.

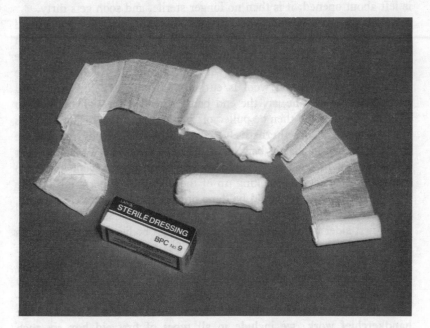

Figure 2.2   Official sterilised individual dressing: boxed; unboxed; open. Note the pad attached to the roller bandage – this must not be touched during application

This is an excellent true first aid dressing for any wound which is at all extensive or is bleeding much, as a preliminary to treatment by a trained nurse, doctor or hospital. As a dressing for small injuries to keep on while at work it is much too bulky. For burns we advise the use of the non-medicated simple sterilised individual dressing.

The official minimum supplies of sterilised individual dressings are shown in Table 2.1.

For further notes and comments on the contents of boxes, look at Chapter 16, *The legal framework*.

Cotton wool (recommended)

Boxes should contain a 'sufficient' supply of absorbent cotton wool in ½ oz (15 g) packets. Cotton wool in substantial quantity is occasionally needed by the first aider for padding a splint, or mopping up a lot of blood. For such purposes, the ½ oz packets have the great merits of cleanliness and convenience. We therefore suggest that each type of first aid box should contain six of these packets. The disadvantage of the ½ oz packet is that this quantity is far too much for most single jobs, for example, cleaning a wound. In consequence, the remainder of a package is left about opened; it is then no longer sterile, and soon gets dirty.

Small pledgets or pieces of cotton wool are essential for wound cleansing. For this purpose, a cotton wool strip dispenser, as used in barber's saloons, is very useful. The model used at Harlow is made from a screw-top jam jar (420 ml) with a ½ inch (1.3 cm) hole cut in the metal top. Clean cotton wool is cut into a ¾ inch (2 cm) strip, and packed neatly into the jar, the end being threaded through the hole in the top. Pledgets can then be pulled off as required. Most major chemists stock dispensers, or, alternatively, cotton wool balls ready for use are available either in plastic bags or in cardboard boxes. We advise that every type of first aid box should contain clean cotton wool in a strip dispenser. The regular stocking up of the dispenser is not a job for the floor of the factory. It should be done on a clean table, in a clean room, by a person with clean hands, preferably a trained nurse.

If a first aider is to attempt to remove foreign bodies from the eye (this question will be discussed in detail later (*see* page 132)), cotton wool is needed in one other form. The 'individual applicator' consists of a wisp of clean cotton wool wound round an orange stick and stored in an envelope. This is a permissible alternative to the corner of the none-too-clean pocket handkerchief, which is still far too common. To discourage handkerchief work, we include in all types of first aid box six such applicators in an envelope, each to be used once and thrown away.

Adhesive plaster (statutory)

The 1981 regulations require a sufficient supply of individually wrapped adhesive plasters in all boxes. Adhesive plaster is used in two forms:

- Individual small plasters, with a gauze dressing attached. Many excellent proprietary varieties are available in different shapes and sizes.
- Reels of plaster, from which strips are cut as required. These strips are not normally applied directly to wounds, but are used to hold other dressings in place.

In our experience, every type of first aid box must contain a large tin of individually wrapped adhesive plaster dressings, preferably in three sizes. So useful and time-saving are these in the treatment of small cuts that, if they are not provided, workers will produce them for themselves.

We prefer the non-water-proof to the water-proof plaster. On a dirty job, the individual small plaster may require frequent changing. Rather than do this, it may be better to cover the plaster with a short length of ordinary bandage, which can then be changed as often as necessary.

A reel of sticking plaster is worth its place in the first aid box, though it should never be applied directly to a wound without some kind of

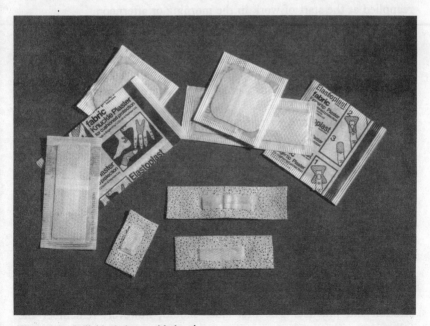

Figure 2.3 Individual plaster with dressing

dressing between it and the injury. Its great value is, as mentioned above, in securing ordinary bandage ends in place.

Protection from oil and solvents

In many jobs, it is necessary to protect a wound from oil, particularly cutting oil. Oil is not necessarily germ-infected; indeed some cutting oils contain an added antiseptic. Nevertheless, oils must be kept away from wounds to prevent their affecting the raw tissues, for this may lead to the development of skin sensitivity later. Oil also delays healing.

The obvious step would appear to be to cover the wound or the dressing with some oil- and waterproof barrier. The barrier has to be waterproof, as many lubricating fluids have a watery basis. To achieve this, rubber fingerstalls and gloves, waterproof plasters, and self-sealing crêpe rubber dressing covers have been tried. With one or two possible exceptions, these all have the serious disadvantage that they retain perspiration, producing a soggy skin around the wound, and so delay healing. Moreover, fingerstalls can be positively dangerous when working with moving machinery. A waterproof plaster should remain on only when the patient is actually at work. It should be removed on leaving work in the evening, and preferably also at the lunch break, and reapplied at the start of work in the morning or afternoon.

Provided it is properly applied and frequently changed, the best protection against oil is an ordinary roller bandage applied over some other dressing. It will need changing at least three times a day – at the start of work and at the end of the morning and afternoon shifts. An oily bandage left in contact with damaged skin overnight predisposes to oil acne and dermatitis.

Special coloured and waterproof plaster dressings are advised for food-handlers and canteen workers. These contain a small metal strip so that the plaster can be detected if lost. Bandages should never be used by such workers.

Roller bandage (recommended)

Roller bandages are not included in the official list of contents, even though they are very useful as coverings for dressings.

Dos and don'ts
The proper use of the roller bandage can be taught only by demonstration and practice. The first aider should, however, remember the following points:

1   Clean the hands before breaking the paper seal.
2   Break the paper by grasping in both hands and contra-rotating (*see* Fig. 2.4).
3   Always work with the bandage rolled.
4   Keep the coil of unused bandage close to the part being bandaged and pull firm after each turn. There is a difference between pulling *firm*, and pulling *tight* – which can be taught only by demonstration and learnt by practice.
5   Do not apply too much bandage.
6   The correct way of tying a bandage must also be taught by demonstration. The bandage end is nicked with scissors, split for about a foot and knotted once to prevent further splitting. Bandages round the

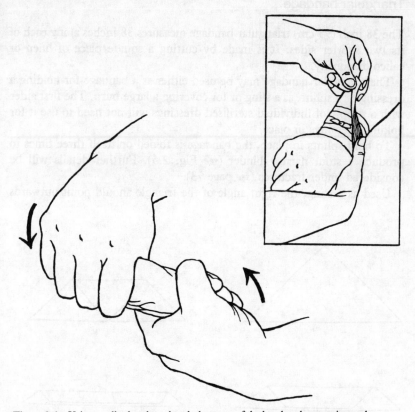

Figure 2.4   Using a roller bandage: break the cover of the bandage by grasping and contra-rotating the hands; (inset) cover the knot and ends of the bandage with adhesive plaster to prevent catching them on moving machinery

fingers, hand or forearm will usually be tied. Bandages round the arm or leg will usually be fixed with a safety pin.

7   Tie the split bandage ends, preferably with a *reef knot*, and cut the ends short to prevent their catching in machinery. The knot and ends are then best covered with a piece of adhesive plaster (*see* Fig. 2.4).

8   Unused roller bandage should be fixed with a pin, and carefully preserved for future use.

There are special methods of bandaging the knee and elbow, shoulder and ankle, scalp, ear and eye. In our view, the first aider will never have to undertake these complicated manoeuvres. These types of injury will usually be dealt with by using a sterilised individual dressing and the patient will then be referred for further treatment to a nurse or doctor.

Triangular bandage

The 38 inch (95 cm) triangular bandage measures 38 inches along each of its two shorter sides. It is made by cutting a square piece of linen or calico diagonally.

The triangular bandage may be used either as a bandage for holding a dressing or a splint, as a sling or for covering a large burn. The first aider with a supply of individual sterilised dressings will not need to use it for holding dressings in place.

To hold splints in place, the bandage is folded on itself three times to produce a stout narrow binder (*see* Fig. 2.5). Further details will be considered under fractures (*see* page 73).

Used as a sling, the right angle of the triangle should point outwards

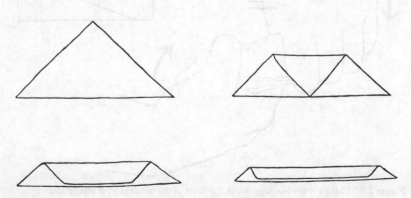

Figure 2.5   Folding a triangular bandage on itself three times to produce a stout narrow binder

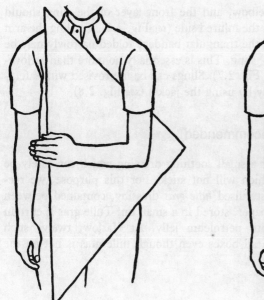
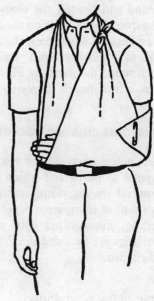

Figure 2.6 The triangular bandage used as a sling: note that the right angle of the triangle points outwards beyond the injured elbow and that the front layer of the sling passes over the shoulder on the injured side

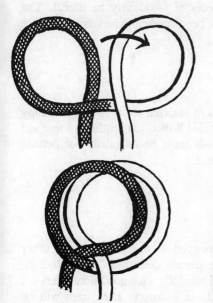
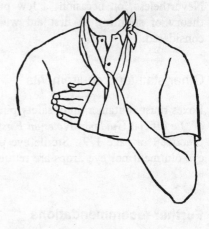

Figure 2.7 The triangular bandage used as a clove hitch: (top) how to make a clove hitch; (bottom) the triangular bandage folded narrow and used as a collar and cuff sling. The cuff is a clove hitch

behind and beyond the elbow, and the front layer of the sling should pass over the shoulder on the injured side (*see* Fig. 2.6). To sling the arm at an angle of 45 degrees, the triangular bandage folded narrowly may be used as a 'collar-and-cuff' sling. This is essentially no more than a clove-hitch round the wrist (*see* Fig. 2.7). Slings can be improvised with safety-pins, a neck-tie, or simply by using the jacket (*see* Fig. 2.8).

Tulle gras dressing (recommended)

First aiders often ask for a small soothing dressing which can safely be applied to burns and which will not stick. For this purpose, we recommend the individual sterilised *tulle gras* dressing, contained between two slips of transparent paper, stored in a small tin. Tulle gras is curtain netting, impregnated with petroleum jelly. At Harlow, twelve such dressings are included in all boxes even though tulle gras is not on the official list.

Splints (recommended)

By law 'suitable splints' with cotton wool or other padding used to be included in the larger boxes. These are not now required. Splints are easy to improvise, and often the best splint is the human body itself. Nevertheless, on occasion, a few pieces of wood may be useful. The theory of splinting in first aid will be discussed when fractures are considered.

Other statutory requirements

Boxes must contain a tin of safety pins of assorted sizes, as well as a copy of the official *Guidance Notes on First Aid* leaflet – an outline of first aid practice (*see* page 179). Sterile eye pads must be included, but neither eye ointment nor eye drops are required.

Further recommendations

To carry out the treatments recommended in this book certain other items are needed in addition to those already described (*see* Table 2.2). In compiling this list, we have studied carefully what good first aiders are already doing and are expected to do in industry. Each item will be discussed in later chapters. Remember that any supplementary items should be authorised by an occupational health nurse or by a doctor. In particular, analgesics, such as aspirin and paracetamol, can only be administered by a first aider under supervision. Even simple medicaments such as throat tablets and preparations for indigestion should be authorised by a trained sister or doctor.

Table 2.2 Supplementary items recommended by Harlow Industrial Health Service

	Number of employees		
	1–11	11–50	51–100
Cotton-wool dispenser containing cotton-wool strip	1	1	1
Individual cotton-wool applicators for eye foreign bodies, in an envelope	6	6	6
Roller bandages, 1 in (2.5 cm × 5 m)	6	9	12
Roller bandages, 2 in (5 cm × 5 m)	6	9	12
Individual sterilised tulle gras dressings, in a tin	12	12	12
Hibitane 0.05 per cent or cetrimide, 1 per cent, in 5, 10 or 20 oz (125, 250 or 500 ml) bottles (depending on space available in box)	10 oz	20 oz	20 oz
Gallipot, plastic, 2 oz (50 ml), now optional	1	1	1
Roll of adhesive plaster (1.3 cm)	1	1	1
Kidney dish, plastic, 6 in (15 cm)	1	1	1
Non-inflammable plaster remover, one 2 oz (50 ml) bottle	1	1	1
Small unbreakable tumbler	1	1	1
Blunt-nosed surgical scissors with chain attached	1	1	1
Splinter forceps	1	1	1
Clinical thermometer, optional.	1	1	1
Tablets (*when recommended by nurse or doctor*):			
Aspirin or paracetamol 0.3 g	12	12	12
Throat tablets	12	12	12
Powder: Compound Magnesium Trisilicate (BPC)	50 g	50 g	50 g

For the protection of first aiders, disposable gloves and apron, household bleach (used with care and according to the manufacturer's instructions) surgical spirit and plastic bags for the disposal of dressings and swabs are recommended. Absorbant paper towels or tissues for mopping up can also be included.

It should be mentioned here that, after use, the kidney-dish, tumbler and gallipot should *always* be washed thoroughly with soap and hot water and dried on a clean towel. If this is not done, infection may be spread from patient to patient.

A note on skin-cleansing agents

We recommend inclusion of a skin-cleansing agent such as cetrimide or hibitane although, officially, this is not required. This is because, officially, first aid is still looked upon as a preliminary to further expert treatment. This is sound enough for anything more than minor injury. But the great bulk of industrial first aid is concerned with minor injury, and most small cuts in industry, as in the home, are never seen by a nurse or a doctor.

It is, however, officially accepted that an adhesive wound dressing will not stick to oily skin. Accordingly, it is suggested that the oil around the wound should be wiped off with cotton wool before an adhesive plaster is applied. In our experience, this is far less satisfactory than using cetrimide or hibitane which we therefore include in the box. (*See further* page 38).

What to leave out

Unless there is a firm discipline and in spite of the official restrictions, many other items soon find their way into the first aid box. The result is an inefficient clutter, with the essentials for sound work lost in a jungle of inessentials. We therefore strongly urge the omission of all items not on the prescribed list. In particular, we regard the following as unnecessary.

Do not include:

- lint, gauze or dressings other than those specified above;
- proprietary or other antiseptics;
- acriflavine solution, cream, emulsion or proprietary preparations;
- mechanically-operated eye-bath and bottle;
- eye lotions, pharmacopoeial or proprietary;

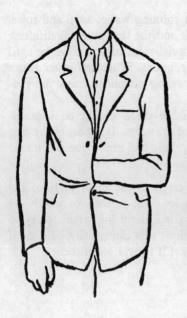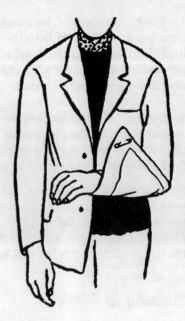

Figure 2.8   The jacket used as an improvised sling

- ointments, pharmacopoeial or proprietary;
- mixtures for internal consumption;
- tablets, other than those specified above;
- styptics;
- lotions for external application.

Many of these items have, in the hands of a doctor or nurse, a proper role in industrial medicine. Before they are used, however, decisions as to diagnosis which are beyond the proper scope of the first aider must be made.

Siting the first aid box

Ideally, the following points should be considered when deciding the situation of the first aid box.

1 *Table*: the box should be fixed to the wall over a small enamel-topped table, which should be kept clear and clean.
2 *Chair*: there should be a strong chair close at hand, on which the patient may sit while being treated.

3 *Water*: there should be a sink, with running water, soap and towel close by, for the use of both the patient and the first aider. A drinking fountain is better than nothing; it has special value in that it can be used for washing out the eye after chemical splashes. When tap water is not available sterile water or saline in disposable containers must be provided.

4 *Disposal of dressings*: beneath the table there should be a pedal-controlled bucket for the disposal of used dressings. It is part of the first aider's job to see that this is emptied regularly and kept clean and lined.

5 *Lighting*: the light should be good.

Sometimes the first aid box will be located in the main body of the workplace, sometimes in a special room set aside partially or wholly for the purpose. If on the shopfloor, it is particularly important to try to preserve a small clear working-space below; this can usually be done if the box is in the stores but it is less easy if it is over a workbench.

Stocking up

In an organised industrial health service, regular inspection and stocking up of first aid boxes is part of the duty of the trained nursing staff. The frequency with which this has to be done will depend on the number of casualties treated. In the Harlow Industrial Health Service, for example, factories are divided into those to be visited weekly, monthly or three-monthly, depending on size and casualty rates. These visits for inspection and stocking help to build a useful link between first aiders and the trained industrial nurses. If stocks run low between visits, first aiders are responsible for letting this be known.

Complaints about the possibility of pilfering from first aid boxes are usually much louder than the facts justify. First-aid boxes should *never* be kept locked; first aid which is delayed while a key is searched for is a travesty. Normally, only a trained first aider should have recourse to the box. It follows that there should always be at least one trained first aider on every shift. Moreover, one particular first aider must be responsible for the box and its stocks. The names of the person in charge and the deputy should be on the outside of it. Where a first aid box is supplementary to a factory first aid room or medical department, it may be used only when the room or department is shut. In such a case, it is helpful if instructions to patients needing treatment are also displayed on the box.

Keeping records

The law in the UK requires certain records of industrial accidents to be kept, but for the most part, minor accidents are excluded. The first aider in charge of a first aid box or post is, however, wise to keep a complete record of all that happens. Such a record may be kept in an ordinary exercise book, appropriately ruled up; it is called a *Day Book*. The *Day Book* should give the date and the name of the patient, the nature of the injury or condition, the cause if this can be stated, the treatment given, and the disposal (back to work, to factory nurse or doctor, or to own doctor or hospital as the case may be). Simple abbreviations will soon be devised. Writing must be kept to a minimum, or it will soon be neglected. The *Day Book* should be kept near the first aid box. It may need to be protected by a plastic cover.

The *Accident Book* is a special ruled-up book issued by the Secretary of State for Social Security (Form BI 510) with space for over 1,000 entries. It is the statutory duty of the employer to provide this book, but the duty of filling it in rests with the employee or his agent. It is the basis for claims under the Industrial Injuries Act (it is the employee's responsibility to make a claim under the Industrial Injuries Act by applying to the local DHSS office). It is also a notification of the accident to the employer who then has the duty to investigate its circumstances. (*See* page 181 for a list of notifiable accidents.)

It is necessary to record in this book only injuries or industrial illnesses which are likely to lead to time off work. But because it must often be difficult to foretell which injuries are serious and which are not, some employers allow their first aid workers to use the *Accident Book* as a *Day Book*, for which it is well suited. The consumption of accident books is then greatly increased. But the employee's rights are safeguarded, and the employer is guaranteed a full picture of what is happening at each first aid post.

All accidents involving more than three days off work, and certain specified serious accidents, have to be notified to either the District Health and Safety Inspector (factories, building sites and farms) or the local Environmental Health Department (shops, offices and restaurants) on Form 2508. A record also has to be kept and the Inspector notified of certain special types of accident, whether or not anyone has been injured. These include crane accidents, explosions, and the collapse of buildings. Details can be found in the leaflet HSE II (Rev). A list of the serious accidents that have to be notified is given in Chapter 16.

Certain industrially caused diseases have also to be recorded and notified to the appropriate authority (as above), this time on Form

2508A. Details are given in leaflet HSE 17. The list of notifiable diseases is also included in Chapter 16.

Leaflets HSE 11 and HSE 17 can be obtained free of charge from:

Public Enquiry Point,
St Hugh's House,
Stanley Precinct,
Bootle,
Merseyside
L20 3QY.

Precautions for first aiders against AIDS and hepatitis B

Due to rising concern over the dangers of certain diseases, particularly AIDS (acquired immune deficiency syndrome), all first aiders should be aware at the outset of any first aid course of risks involved in treatment of wounds and the precautions to be taken.

Infection

The viruses causing the diseases AIDS and hepatitis B are found in the blood and semen of those patients suffering from, or carrying the infections. The diseases can only be passed on to another person by the direct introduction of the virus into their blood stream. In practice, this means that infection can only occur through sexual intercourse, or by contamination of an open wound by infected blood.

Risk of infection

A first aider, treating an infected patient suffering from a bleeding wound could only be at risk if he or she had a cut or abrasion on the hand, or had cut or pricked him or herself on an instrument or needle contaminated with the patient's blood.

The number of people who are aids or hepatitis B carriers is still *very small* in most parts of the country. Anyone who knows they are a carrier ought to be encouraged to inform first aiders (and, of course, medical and nursing staff), if they require first aid treatment for an injury. Should they do so, *the first aider must treat such information as completely confidential* (as with any personal information given). He or she must reassure all patients that nothing will be passed on without the patient's permission.

It is, however, possible that patients, knowing themselves to be carriers of AIDS or hepatitis B, are either afraid to admit this to medical staff or management, or are unaware of their condition.

The first aider could, in these circumstances be at risk without realising it, and would not be in a position to assess any risk unless working under the guidance of a nurse or doctor. Even though any risk is extremely small, especially when treating the vast majority of minor injuries, it is advisable to get into the habit of taking routine precautions, following the same guidelines with every patient, so that there is no suggestion of discrimination against any one individual.

These precautions are outlined below.

Guidelines for protection against AIDS and hepatitis B

These guidelines are only simple hygiene rules to help prevent the spread of any contact infection; most of them are recommended in this book. Very few additional precautions are needed to give extra protection against AIDS and hepatitis B.

Antiseptics

The best general antiseptic for disinfection against these diseases is household bleach, diluted two teaspoons of bleach in one pint (½ litre) of water. This cannot be used for cleaning wounds, but it can be used for cleaning bench tops, sink units, and anything that has been in contact with blood. Any virus is probably killed within a minute and definitely within ten minutes. *Remember that bleach is very irritant to the skin and to the eyes.* Gloves should be worn when wiping down and care taken to avoid splashes into the eyes, preferably by wearing safety spectacles. Any splashes should be immediately washed off with running water as described later in the book.

It is recommended that a bottle of household bleach be kept in every first aid room or treatment area with a plastic jug or bowl in which to dilute it (it will attack metal). The provision of protective gloves is now required under the Regulations, (in case the patient is contaminated with a chemical), and a pair of safety spectacles is a sensible addition to any first aid facility.

Hygiene rules for treating bleeding wounds

1 The first aider should always cover *all* cracks, cuts and abrasions on his or her hands with a *waterproof plaster*, after washing well with soap and water, and drying with a clean towel. A first aider will, of course, treat any minor wounds on his or her own hands as described in the next chapter on wound treatment. No first aider should undertake any

treatment of patients if he or she has any wounds which are too large to be covered by the standard size adhesive plaster, or if he or she is suffering from dermatitis or eczema of the hands.

2   If these precautions are difficult, or if the first aider prefers, light weight, disposable gloves can be worn. These should be changed after each patient.

3   After treatment, all used surfaces, and all plastic dishes, should be wiped down with paper towels or tissues soaked in household bleach, diluted two teaspoons bleach in one pint (½ litre) of water. Leave for ten minutes before washing down with plain water.

4   All blood-stained dressings, disposable gloves and paper towels used for wiping down should be placed in a plastic bag which can be tied at the top and so sealed before disposal.

5   The first aider should then wash his or her own hands in soap and water and change any dressings.

6   If the first aider accidently contaminates any open wound with blood it should immediately be washed with running water making it bleed at the same time. The wound is best treated with surgical spirit, 70%, applied either by swabbing with cotton wool or by soaking the wound in spirit for five minutes. In the case of a superficial cut or abrasion this treatment will kill off any infection. In the case of a puncture wound or deep cut, unlikely in first aid practice, the accident should be reported to a nurse or doctor for further advice. The most valuable part of the treatment is to encourage early bleeding from the wound. The risk to a first aid worker who follows these guidelines, is negligible.

Surgical spirit is therefore another recommended addition to the first aid equipment, *not for the routine treatment of wounds, but solely for emergency use as described above*. It would be especially useful to carry in mobile packs when first aid treatment might have to be given where no running water is available.

Mouth-to-mouth resuscitation
The methods of resuscitation are described later in the book (*see* page 115). Complete protection can be provided by the use of a plastic protector:

1   *Resusci Ade*, a plastic mouth piece, obtainable from:

Portex Ltd,
Hythe, Kent.

This can also be disinfected by soaking in bleach (two teaspoons bleach to one pint water), preferably for ten minutes, followed by thorough rinsing in water. It is probably better though to treat it as disposable.

2   Laerdal Pocket mask: this is a transparent plastic mask made to fit over the patient's nose and mouth. It can be obtained from:

Laerdal Medical Ltd
Laerdal House
Goodmead Rd
Orpington, Kent

It is *not* disposable and must be cleaned as described above.

3   Bioglan Microshield: a very effective plastic mouth piece, obtainable from:

Bioglan Laboratories Ltd
1 The Cam Centre
Wilbury Way
Hitchen, Herts SG4   OTW

Manikins
All manikins used for practice should be dismantled, according to the manufacturer's instructions and disinfected in exactly the same way as described above.

Note

It must be emphasised again that AIDS and Hepatitis B cannot be caught either from direct contact or from exhaled breath or droplet infection. There must be direct blood to blood contact, or contact through sexual intercourse.

Review questions

1   Describe the dressings that must be provided by law in every first aid box in any workplace and explain their use.
2   How would you protect yourself against the risk of infection from AIDS or any other blood-born disease?

3   Wounds and the control of bleeding

Definitions

We define a wound as any break in the skin, with or without injury to the deeper tissues. Thus, the term *wound* covers every type of skin break, from the trivial scratch to the severe crush injury.

The skin is the body tissue most liable to injury, and it is estimated that in Britain every day there are half a million skin injuries of sufficient size to need at least a first aid dressing. Of these, one in every ten needs attention at a factory or health centre.

It follows that wounds are by far the commonest reason for first aid. Experienced first aiders will have treated many different types of wound. Even beginners must have seen cuts of various kinds. It is a useful class exercise for each member to describe a wound he or she has seen and how it was caused.

Here are some examples of typical wounds that occur at work:

1   **Incised wound**: e.g. a straight cut from a chisel or sheet metal.
2   **Lacerated wound**: e.g. a tearing wound with ragged edges where flesh has, perhaps, been caught in a machine.
3   **Contused wound**: e.g. a crushing wound with the flesh around bruised and injured from a hammer-blow, or injury from a spanner or rollers.
4   **Puncture wound**: e.g. a deep stab, from stepping on a nail. Incidentally, a severe puncture wound may bleed very little or may not even bleed at all.
5   **Abrasion**: e.g. a scraping wound or graze, where the skin surface it torn by a file or sandpaper, for example.

Identifying major and minor wounds

The most important division for all first aiders to learn, especially in industrial first aid, is the distinction between major and minor wounds.

- Minor or simple wounds – the ordinary everyday small skin cuts which can properly be treated by the first aider.
- Major wounds – everything more severe than the minor wound. For these the first aider gives true first aid treatment only, pending the arrival of, or referral to, a trained nurse or a doctor.

This division of wounds emphasises the most important single decision which the industrial first aider has to make.

- Can I properly treat this wound myself?
- Ought I to apply first aid only and send for, or refer to, a trained nurse or doctor?

The first aider must never feel reluctant about passing on the patient to more skilled hands – just as the nurse passes the patient on to the general practitioner, and the general practitioner passes on to the specialist. The good first aider thinks only of the patient's welfare and so is always ready to seek further help. The inept first aider tries to be an amateur doctor, to the danger of the patient, and at some legal risk to the employer and him or herself.

In the case of obviously severe wounds, there is no difficulty in making a decision; nor is there any with the half-inch long shallow graze on the hand. Between these two there are many types of wound where the first aider in industry will have to make a judgment. There are three things to be considered:

- The position
- The type of wound
- Complications

The position of the wound

1 Any wound around the eye or involving the skin of the face is serious.
2 Any wound, other than a small shallow cut, of the finger, hand or wrist is to be treated as serious; even a small scar on a finger may reduce the skill and affect the livelihood of a manual worker.
3 Any wound of the abdomen is serious.

The type of wound

1 Any wound with ragged edges or with the flesh around it bruised is serious, because the damaged tissue is more liable to infection.
2 Any deep wound or stab or puncture wound is serious, because infection can be carried in by the wounding object, and because there may be unseen damage to deeper tissues.

3   Any gaping wound, the edges of which do not easily come together, is serious, because the exposed raw area is more likely to get infected, and the scar will be wide and disabling.

Complications of the wound
1   Any wound from which the blood pumps out in jerks is serious, because this means an artery has been cut.
2   Any wound from which the blood gushes out in a steady stream is serious because this means a vein has been cut.
3   Any wound more than an eighth of an inch deep may involve damage to muscles, tendons, nerves or other structures. This risk is greatest in the wrist, hand and fingers. The first aider cannot tell if these structures have been injured.

Bleeding or haemorrhage

Bleeding (haemorrhage) is part of the natural response to injury so it need not cause alarm in the first aider or the patient. Bleeding is nature's means of wound cleansing: it washes dirt out from the bottom of the wound.

Too much bleeding, however, is a danger, simply because, beyond a certain point, the body cannot swiftly make up for blood loss, but bleeding from *most* wounds will stop spontaneously without any treatment at all (*see* Fig. 3.1).

Stopping bleeding

The body has two very effective methods of stopping bleeding:

1   the clotting of blood, as a result of its coming in contact with cut and injured tissues;
2   the pulling back and shrinking of the cut ends of blood vessels, so that the holes from which the blood is coming get smaller and may close entirely.

Bleeding from *minor* wounds will occur during the cleansing of the wound; it helps to make the cleansing more thorough. As soon as the wound is covered and the edges drawn together by the dressing, clotting of the blood will take place and the bleeding will stop.

Bleeding from *major* wounds will also usually stop on its own when a dressing is applied. The first aider can do three things to help the body to stop such bleeding:

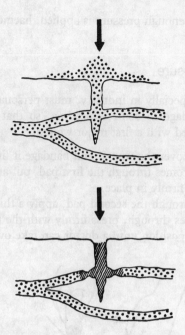

Figure 3.1 How the body stops bleeding: (top) at the moment of wounding blood pours from the cut vessels; (bottom) within a few minutes the blood has clotted to form a tough jelly and the cut ends of the blood vessels have pulled back and shrunk. (Fluid blood is shown as dots and clotted blood as lines; the arrows show the site of the wound)

- Let the patient rest
- Raise the injured part
- Apply pressure

Rest
Make the patient lie down quietly, and keep the wounded part still. This lowers the blood pressure and slows the pulse, so that the volume of blood flowing through the injured part is lessened.

Raising the injured part
If the injured part is raised above the level of the rest of the body, the amount of blood reaching it will be less. A wounded arm or leg may be raised by pillows, but the stomach or chest cannot be effectively raised.

Pressure on the place which is bleeding
This is the most important and effective way of controlling bleeding. It

can be stated that if enough pressure is applied, haemorrhage can always be controlled.

How to apply pressure

Every first aider, especially in industry, must personally practise applying a pad and bandage to control bleeding, so that this can be done effectively when faced with a first major wound.

- Place a clean pad over the wound and bandage it firmly in place.
- If blood quickly comes through the first pad, put another pad on top, and bandage this firmly in place.
- If blood comes through the second pad, apply a third pad.
- If blood still comes through, press firmly with the hands on the third pad, and hold in position until a doctor can take over (*see* Fig. 3.2).

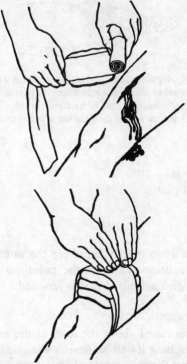

Figure 3.2 Stopping severe bleeding: (top) applying a pad and bandage (sterilised individual dressing) to stop haemorrhage; (bottom) if, after three pads have been applied, the blood still comes through, the last pad must be pressed upon firmly until medical help arrives. At the same time, the leg should be raised above the horizontal position

As already stressed, sterilised individual dressing is ideal for the control of bleeding, since it has a built-in pad attached to a bandage, and the whole dressing is sterilised. If an official first aid dressing is not available, a rolled-up bandage may be used as a pad, or a clean folded handkerchief. If necessary, a clean handkerchief may also be used as a bandage.

Never look for pressure points

In the past most first aiders were taught that there are certain points between the heart and the site of bleeding where, by pressing hard against an underlying bone, the arterial flow can be stopped. Most doctors, however, never make use of these pressure points and we recommend the abandonment of pressure point teaching in first aid. We do not expect any first aider to risk the patient's life by hunting for a pressure point instead of applying direct pressure to the place which is actually bleeding.

Never attempt to make a tourniquet

First aid boxes should never contain a rubber or pressure bandage for use as a tourniquet. A tourniquet should never be used, as it is not a first aid measure. It is often ineffective and frequently harmful. If properly applied, it can cause death of a limb. If improperly applied, it can increase bleeding by obstructing the veins but not the arteries. Finally, it is *never* necessary, as bleeding can always be stopped by the safe simple method of direct pressure.

Deep cuts of wrist or arm

Such a cut, particularly at the wrist, may produce spirting or pumping haemorrhage if one of the larger arteries is cut. If this happens, treatment follows exactly the lines set out above. Again:

1 make the patient lie down;
2 hold up the arm, so as to raise the injured part above the level of the rest of body;
3 place a clean pad over the wound, and bind it very firmly in place. Apply another pad and bandage;
4 send for a trained nurse or doctor, or transport the patient to the health centre or hospital. If possible, the patient should be lying down, with the arm and wrist raised on a pillow or folded blanket.

Blood loss

About one-eleventh of the weight of the body is blood. There are about 12 pints (6.5 litres) of blood in the average adult. A little blood can make a big mess; to demonstrate this, upset a two-ounce (50 ml) bottle of red ink and see how much bandage and cotton wool it will colour. A normal adult can lose a pint of blood without ill effect; many people give this much blood twice a year to the blood transfusion service. Most bleeding is not serious, and the first aider need never be frightened by it.

On the other hand, the loss of a large amount of blood produces a very dangerous state. As the bleeding goes on, it leads to pallor and weakness, then unconsciousness and can finally result in death. If life is to be saved, after the bleeding has been controlled by firm pressure, it is vital at the earliest possible moment to replace the blood which has been lost, by means of a blood transfusion.

A patient who is believed to have lost a large amount of blood must be moved as swiftly as possible to a hospital where a blood transfusion can be started at once.

Blood transfusion

If transfusion can be started within half an hour, life will probably be saved; delay of over an hour may prove fatal. By making arrangements quickly and calmly, the first aider is acting in a life-saving role.

It will help the doctor at the hospital to estimate the amount of blood which has been lost, and hence the amount of blood the patient needs, if the blood lost can be mopped or scooped up, and the blood and stained dressings, cotton wool and clothing put in an enamel basin and sent with the patient to hospital. But do not waste time on this if it means delay in getting the patient there.

Cover the patient with two blankets or a coat. Apart from lifting out of danger or on to a stretcher, keep movement to a minimum.

Infection of wounds

Infection is the entry of harmful germs into a wound so that they start to grow and multiply.

Every year too many workers suffer from infected injuries, and each could lose several weeks of working time. Even minor degrees of infection can involve about three days off work. Clearly, the prevention of infection in first aid is just as important as the control of bleeding.

Germs get carried into a wound by whatever causes the wound – a nail, hammer, chisel, cutting tool, drill or knife. Even if the injuring instrument is germ-free, for example a very hot tool, germs may be picked up as it passes through the patient's boot or shoe, clothing and skin. These germs are got rid of by the process of cleaning the wound, and, as already mentioned, by bleeding.

After the original injury, germs may still get in by droplet-spray infection, from people talking, sneezing or coughing near the wound, or from the skin or careless first aiders, doctors or nurses. These germs are kept out by surgical cleaning techniques and by closing and covering the wound.

When germs were first discovered, doctors sought chemical substances which would kill them. Such chemical substances are called antiseptics. Unfortunately, most antiseptics not only kill germs; they also damage human tissues. In addition, they may sometimes produce skin rashes. For these reasons, their use as a means of trying to kill germs in wounds has been largely given up. In fact, in modern first aid:

Iodine and other tissue-damaging antiseptics have no place and should not under any circumstances be poured into or on a wound.

Cleaning the wound

Major wounds

A *major* wound needs thorough cleaning by a trained nurse or doctor. An extensive major wound may need opening and cleaning thoroughly by a surgeon, with the patient or at least the wounded part anaesthetised. Delay in getting a major wound properly cleaned increases the likelihood of the germs gaining a foothold in the tissues. The first aider's job is to cover the major wound with a sterile pad as quickly as possible.

Minor wounds

A *minor* wound is best cleaned by washing thoroughly with clean water under a running tap (*see* Fig. 3.3). If there is any visible dirt present around the minor wound, it may be washed away with soap and water. Better even than soap are the cleaning agents hibitane and cetrimide (*Cetavlon*); these have both a detergent and an antiseptic action and do not injure the tissues.

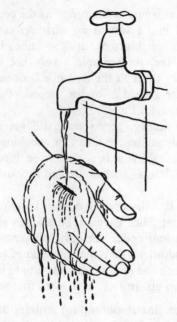

Figure 3.3   Cleaning a minor wound under a tap: a minor wound is best cleaned simply by washing thoroughly with clean water under a running tap

How to clean a wound

In cleaning or covering a minor wound, the first aider must take all reasonable steps to keep germs away from the cleaned wound and the dressing. Ideally, hands should be washed thoroughly before starting cleaning or dressing, but in some workplaces this may be impossible. The first aider must be careful not to cough, sneeze or talk over the wound. Even more important is to keep his or her own skin germs away from the wound or anything which is going to touch the wound surface. This means no touching of the wound with the fingers, and no touching of the surface of the dressing which will be placed next to the wound. Every first aider must practise this simplified *no-touch* method of dressing wounds until it is quite automatic.

In many workplaces, running water is not available at the first aid point. Here, cleaning of the wound and surrounding skin is best done with cotton wool dipped in hibitane or cetrimide or with the sterile water or saline that must be available, with soap if necessary. (*See* Fig. 3.4).

(a) Wash the hands thoroughly.
(b) Pour the solution into a kidney dish or small gallipot.

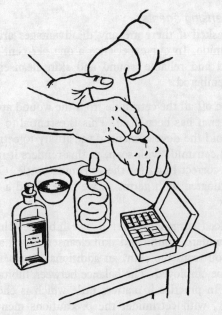

Figure 3.4 Cleaning a minor wound without running water. If running water is not available at the first aid point the standard method recommended of cleaning a minor wound is to use cotton wool swabs dipped in hibitane (0.05 per cent) or cetrimide (one per cent), or sterile water or saline with soap. A kidney dish is a satisfactory substitute for the gallipot shown in the figure. The bottle should have a screw cap

(c) Dip a piece of cotton wool (about two inches long) into the solution.

(d) Clean the wound thoroughly.

(e) Repeat this process twice more with fresh cotton wool each time.

(f) Clean the skin around the wound in a similar way, taking care to work outwards from the wound. Avoid touching the wound with the cotton wool used for skin cleaning.

(g) Dry first the wound then the surrounding skin thoroughly with fresh dry pieces of cotton wool so as to remove all the solution (or soap and water). This is necessary for two reasons:

(i) hibitane, cetrimide or soap left in contact with raw tissue may lead to sensitivity, with the possibility of a skin rash later on;

(ii) unless the skin is dry, strapping will not stick to it.

(h) After use throw each piece of cotton wool into an appropriate receptacle (such as a lined bin).

(i) Cover the wound with an appropriately-sized adhesive plaster dressing so that the edges of the wound are drawn together.

Using skin-cleansing agents

We are often asked if there are any disadvantages arising out of such agents as cetrimide. In our experience a one per cent solution of cetrimide is a good and reliable wound and skin cleanser, provided three points are remembered:

1   Always wipe off all the cetrimide from the wound and skin with clean cotton wool after it has been used. This is essential to get the plaster to stick and to avoid the development of sensitivity to cetrimide.
2   Do not mix cetrimide with soap, as this renders it inactive.
3   Choose the correct bung for the cetrimide bottle. Corks are liable to become contaminated with germs so we have found a plastic screw cap the best answer.

Many experienced surgeons prefer to use hibitane (chlorhexidine) 0.05 per cent as a standard wound and skin cleanser in first aid. If this fails to remove heavy oil from the skin, an additional cleanser such as Zoff or Swarfega may be employed. The balance between hibitane and cetrimide is a close one. In practice it matters little which is chosen for both are good. However, with cetrimide, the precautions mentioned above are essential.

Closing and covering the wound

Any wound which is left gaping is liable to become infected. Even if not infected, a gaping wound will heal much more slowly, and will leave behind a wide and perhaps disabling scar. This is why the first aider must regard any gaping wound as a major wound, to be covered with a clean or sterile dressing and passed on at once to a trained nurse or doctor. Many gaping wounds will require stitching (*suturing*) to bring the edges together, for which most doctors nowadays use a local anaesthetic.

The wound which has been properly cleaned, closed and covered will heal in the shortest possible time, almost without pain, and with the smallest possible scar. In surgery, this is spoken of as *healing by first intention*. It is the object of good first aid, good industrial medicine, and good casualty surgery, to enable every wound to heal by first intention.

A note for first aiders in the food industry or canteens

Under the various Food Hygiene Regulations, workers in the food industries have to keep all cuts and abrasions on exposed parts (that is, the hands, arms and face) covered with a suitable *waterproof* dressing. This provision is met if the assorted adhesive wound dressings in the first aid box are of the waterproof variety.

The first aid worker in such industries will be wise in addition to cover any dressing on the fingers with a waterproof plastic fingerstall secured by tapes around the wrist. This precaution keeps to a minimum the risk of an adhesive dressing coming loose and getting into food in the course of its manufacture or preparation.

The Food Hygiene Regulations also specify that the first aid stocks provided in food industries must include suitable and sufficient *bandages* and *antiseptic*. Neither of these is now included in the official contents of first aid boxes. They are, however, included in the supplement which we recommend. Thus, our boxes will fully cover the statutory requirements in the food industries (*see* Table 2.2).

The regulations also require a notice to be fixed in each lavatory, asking everyone to wash their hands after using the lavatory.

Review questions

1   Describe how you would deal with a small superficial cut on the hand.
2   How would you treat a deep cut on the ankle that was bleeding very badly?

4 Treating wounds

The principles governing the treatment of wounds covered in the last chapter must now be extended to cover wounds of special types and in special places. But first the standard treatment of minor and major wounds must be recapitulated, so that the necessary variations to meet special conditions may be seen in proper relation to standard procedure.

Treating minor wounds

In treating a minor wound the prevention of infection is more important than the control of bleeding. With proper treatment to prevent infection, bleeding will stop on its own. Look again at the stages of treatment – clean, dry, and cover – on page 36.

Dressing minor wounds
Here are a few additional points to note when dressing minor wounds.

1 If the wound is on a part of the body which is continually in movement, such as the hand, or is liable to get soiled with dirt or oil, the strapping should be covered with a *neatly-applied* roller bandage. Even a short end of bandage is a danger to a machine operator. So after the bandage has been split and tied and the ends cut short, these ends should be covered with one or two turns of strapping. The first aider should practise this under supervision, remembering that:

neatness is essential

2 At the beginning and end of each working day, or better still each four-hour working period, a fresh outer bandage should be applied. *It is dangerous to leave soiled and oil-stained bandages over a raw wound for any length of time*, for example, overnight; this is one cause of skin sensitivity and dermatitis.

3 Tubular stretch dressings, such as *tube gauze* are frequently applied

by nurses and doctors, particularly to cover finger injuries. Though excellent in skilled hands these are not recommended for the first aid worker.

4 A bandage gives partial protection only against oil. The alternative – a cover of rubber or similar material to completely enclose the dressing is not recommended. Should such a covering be used, it must never be allowed to stay on for more than a few hours, or the skin beneath it will become soggy. A protective bandage, frequently changed, is to be preferred, since the skin beneath stays in better condition and healing is therefore quicker. Workers in food factories should not use bandages as dressings, to prevent any possible contamination of the product by parts of the bandage coming loose (*see* pg 38).

Re-dressing minor wounds

A minor wound should be re-dressed as seldom as possible. If there is no pain, it is only necessary to change the outer dressing when it is soiled; the dressing immediately over the wound should be left in position, if possible, for 48 hours. Exactly the same care must be used in changing a dressing as when the dressing is first applied.

If the patient complains of pain or discomfort in a minor wound on the day after injury or thereafter, the first aider *must* refer the patient at once to a trained nurse or doctor, as infection is likely to have occurred.

Treating major wounds

Again, treating the major wound is a matter of applying procedures already described. Here the first aider gives true first aid, pending the arrival of, or referral to, a trained nurse or doctor.

The first aider will make no attempt to clean a major wound, but must:

1 prevent any further risk of infection by covering the surface of the wound with a sterile or clean dressing as quickly as possible.

2 control haemorrhage by making the patient lie down quietly, raising the injured part, and binding the pad or dressing over the wound firmly in place.

The ideal pad and bandage is the official individual sterilised first aid dressing. If the bleeding rapidly soaks through, one or more pads should be applied and firmly bound in place over the first one.

Once a major wound has been covered, the sooner expert help is obtained the better for the patient.

Foreign bodies in wounds

A large foreign body, such as a piece of metal or glass, if sticking out of the wound, should be removed gently, provided this can be done without putting the fingers into the wound. If any foreign body does not come out easily, it should be left alone. A note that it has been seen should be sent on with the patient when referred for further treatment.

In a severe injury, there may on rare occasions be a piece of bone projecting through the wound or the skin; this should be left alone and not touched.

Using rolled bandages

If a large foreign body cannot be removed, or if there is projecting bone direct pressure *must not* be applied. Rolled bandages, with the paper removed, may be placed on each side of the projecting object; the wound, object and rolled bandages are then covered with a large individual first aid dressing; this should be bandaged in place firmly but not tightly (*see* Fig. 4.1). Most first aiders are taught to build up a ring or box of dressing around wounds of this type, so that the covering dressing does not press on the wound. But rolled bandages are just as good, and to put them in place takes very little time, reducing the risk of infection.

Bleeding

If there is severe bleeding from a wound in which there is a foreign body, control of the bleeding must take precedence over treatment of the foreign body.

Special wounds

Small crush, graze or laceration

Any crush, graze or laceration, other than a very small one, is to be treated as a major wound and referred to a trained nurse or doctor.

The proper treatment for a really small crush, graze or laceration is thorough cleaning with cetrimide followed by a dry dressing, protected by a bandage to keep it clean (*see* page 36). Anything larger should be covered with a sterilised first aid dressing and referred to a trained nurse or doctor.

Wound of the scalp

Small scalp wounds heal well with no dressing at all. Clean the wound

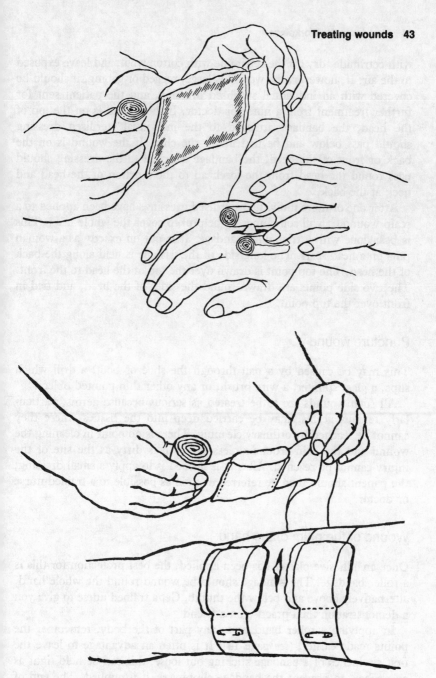

Figure 4.1 Protecting and bandaging a wound to cover a projecting foreign body. Note the
two rolled bandages, held in place by the patient or an assistant, and so arranged as to prevent
the dressing pad from pressing hard on the foreign body when the bandage is fixed; (bottom)
when the projecting foreign body is large the pads of two individual sterilised dressings are
used to relieve pressure

with cetrimide, dry off the cetrimide with cotton wool, and leave exposed to the air. If, however, the wound is large, ragged or gaping, it should be covered with an individual sterilised dressing, and the patient sent for further treatment from a nurse or doctor. If the wound is on the top of the head, the bandage attached to the individual sterilised dressing should pass below and be tied under the chin. If the wound is on the back or front of the head, the bandage attached to the dressing should pass round the head from the forehead to the junction of the head and neck at the back.

After one or more individual sterilised dressings have been applied to a scalp wound, it will sometimes be helpful to cover the whole head. This is best done with a triangular bandage. It is put on exactly as a woman puts on a head scarf. The long side of the triangle is held along the back of the head. The top point is drawn over the top of the head to the front. The two side points are drawn round the sides of the head, and tied in front over the top point.

Puncture wound

This may be caused by a nail through the shoe or boot, a drill which slips, a glass splinter, a wire brush, or any other thin pointed object.

All such wounds are to be treated as serious because germs, particularly tetanus germs, may be carried deep into the tissues where they cannot be reached by ordinary cleaning. There is no point in cleaning the wound and the skin around unless the skin is dirty as the site of the injury cannot be reached. All that is needed is to apply a small dressing; the patient should then be referred as soon as possible to a trained nurse or doctor.

Wound of the palm of the hand

Once an adhesive plaster has been applied, the best protection for this is a roller bandage. The bandage should be wound round the whole hand, alternatively above and below the thumb. Get a trained nurse to give you a demonstration then practise on a friend.

In applying a roller bandage to any part of the body, remember the points made earlier, (*see* page 14). It is often an advantage to leave the first six inches of a bandage sticking out loose; this can be held tight as an anchor, to prevent the bandage slipping as it is applied. The end of the bandage can be tied to this loose piece, to finish off when the application is complete.

Animal or human bite

The mouth is full of germs, so bites are usually badly infected. More-over, they are often also lacerated or puncture wounds. Every bite, however small, should be treated as a major wound, as set out above. (*See also protection against AIDS and hepatitis B on page 24*).

Wound of the chest

A crush wound of the chest may damage the lungs. The patient may cough up blood and find it hard to breathe. Breathing may be easier if the patient is propped up in the semi-sitting position, but what is most important is to find the position of greatest comfort for the patient.

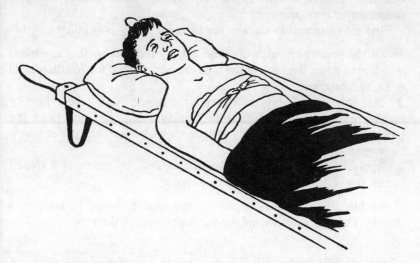

Figure 4.2 Covering a puncture wound of the chest: a large pad and bandage is applied to help keep out the air which tends to be sucked in at each breath. A folded triangular bandage tied round the chest is used to keep the pad firmly in place

A puncture wound of the chest is a rare occurrence. Sometimes the puncture may actually reach into the chest cavity. With such a wound, air is sucked in at each breath. It should be covered at once with a large dressing, which must be fixed on firmly to keep out the air (*see* Fig. 4.2).

Any patient with a chest wound should be moved to hospital as quickly as possible.

Wound of the abdomen

Because of the risk that an abdominal wound may have punctured the stomach or bowels, it is very important that the patient should be given nothing to eat or drink but should be moved to hospital without delay.

Nose bleeding

Epistaxis or nose bleeding may follow a blow on the nose, nose picking or a bad cold; such nose bleeding will usually stop quickly. Or it may follow a severe head injury, which means usually that the skull is fractured. Often nose bleeding is spontaneous and has no obvious external cause; this type is more likely to last for some time and perhaps be serious. It is not part of first aid to attempt to diagnose the cause of spontaneous nose bleeding. If there is other serious injury, its treatment must take precedence over nose bleeding.

First aid treatment in the absence of major injury is as follows:

1   Sit the patient up, with the head slightly forward, so that any blood which runs down the back of the nose can escape from the mouth instead of being swallowed.
2   Make the patient breathe through the mouth (this is best done by making him or her bite on something, for instance a cork), and pinch the nose firmly so that the nostrils are closed. Thereafter, the patient must be warned not to sniff.
3   Apply cold water to the bridge of the nose, by means of a soaked handkerchief or cotton wool soaked in water.

If the bleeding continues or recurs, the patient should be seen by a doctor. The first aider should *never* attempt to plug the nose.

Ruptured varicose veins

A varicose vein is an enlarged leg vein just under the skin in which the blood is circulating inefficiently. Varicose veins are common in both sexes in those over 40.

A small leg wound which penetrates a varicose vein will bleed profusely. Here first aid can be life-saving.

The treatment follows exactly the general principles for all serious bleeding:

1   Rest. The patient should lie down.
2   Raise the wounded part. For example, the foot should be raised, and

when the wound has been dressed, the leg should be supported with cushions or pillows.

3 Direct pressure on the bleeding part. A sterile pad should be applied and firmly bandaged in place. This should stop the bleeding almost at once. One or more pads should be bound on top of the first if necessary.

It is *very dangerous* to apply a tourniquet to a leg with a bleeding varicose vein, as it may increase the haemorrhage.

Stings, insect bites and blisters

Bee and wasp stings may occur at work as elsewhere. They are a special risk in jam factories.

Bees
The *bee* leaves both its sting and poison bag behind. If the sting is grasped with a pair of forceps in order to pull it out, the contents of the poison bag may be pumped into the patient. The sting is best lifted or scraped off the skin with one blade of a pair of forceps or with a pin. The patient should then suck the wound and spit out.

The only other local treatments of any value are:

- the application of a propietary *antihistamine* and calamine ointment;
- applying a cold compress or an ice pack.

If the sting is in the mouth, skilled nursing or medical help is required at once. While help is coming, the patient should be given a piece of ice to suck.

Wasps
The *wasp* leaves no sting behind, so the patient should suck the wound and spit out forthwith. Further local treatment is exactly the same as for a bee sting – antihistamine ointment, a cold compress or an ice pack. As with a bee sting, if the wasp sting is in the mouth, skilled help should be sought at once, and ice given to suck.

With any sting, the patient may start to swell up either around the injury or generally, or show signs of shock. If this happens skilled nursing or medical help is needed immediately.

Spider and snakes
Spider and *snake* bites may occur in industrial workers. Those at risk are dockers and banana-ripening store operatives. The creatures are

imported in banana bunches, usually from Brazil. They are not found in West Indian bananas, though a three-inch non-biting spider is sometimes seen. The Brazilian banana spider is huge, with a two-inch body and a leg span of six or more inches. It is not a true tarantula. Its bite will draw blood but is usually not serious; nevertheless, anyone bitten should be sent to a hospital or doctor.

The snake most often seen is the Brazilian tree snake, but even this is very rare. The treatment is as for other snake bites.

- Wash the bites thoroughly, to remove any venom which the snake may have spat out into the skin.
- Suck the wound hard and spit out.
- Tie a bandage (or the bandage part of a sterilised individual dressing) tightly round the limb, between the bite and the body. This will not stop the blood flow, but will cut down the flow of lymph (body tissue fluid) back to the body; it is in the lymph that the venom mainly travels.
- Loosen the bandage for half a minute every quarter of an hour.
- Send for skilled help at once, or send the patient immediately to hospital.

The snake should be sent in a box with the patient for identification.

Mosquito and other bites
Patients sometimes arrive at work with painful swellings due to *mosquito* or other bites. These are not first aid problems and need nursing or medical examination and care.

Blisters
Blisters, other than blood-blisters, are not emergencies, though they may be very incapacitating. The first aider should not puncture blisters as the chances of carrying in infection are high. The blister and surrounding skin should be cleaned gently with hibitane or cetrimide, and covered with a dry dressing; under this the blister may burst spontaneously and safely. If a blister is painful or obviously infected, it should be seen by a trained nurse or doctor.

Contusions

A *contusion* or bruise is bleeding under the skin, with the skin surface unbroken. First aiders will be able to think of many examples: the bruised bottom, following a slip, a fall downstairs, or a skating accident;

the black eye; the thick ear; the egg-like bruise on the scalp; the bruise on the front of the shin; the bruise under the nail following a pinch from a door or a weight dropped on a toe; the bruise over the ribs.

Faced with a bruise, the main duty of the first aider is to make sure:

(a) that no bones are broken; and
(b) there is no other serious injury. If slight movement causes severe pain, serious injury must be assumed.

Because germs cannot get through the intact skin, no dressing is needed over a bruise. Pain may be relieved by a cold compress, recooled as often as necessary, or by an ice pack. A cold compress is made by dipping a clean folded handkerchief or a folded triangular bandage in water; this is placed on the bruise, without wringing out; it may then be covered with cotton wool and a firm bandage. An ice pack may be made by wrapping ice cubes in a thick towel and crushing them with a mallet.

No attempt should ever be made by a first aider to empty a bruise by puncturing it. The idea that it is necessary to *bring out a bruise* is an old wives' tale.

Review questions

1   How would you deal with a patient with a bleeding nose?
2   A middle-aged lady is bleeding badly from the right leg. What might the trouble be? What would you do?

Also try the questions on treatment of wounds on page 163.

5 Shock and other effects of serious injury

Shock

Every severely injured patient soon develops *shock*. Without proper treatment, shock can be fatal. With proper treatment applied quickly enough, the patient almost always recovers. Proper treatment of shock can be summed up in the words: *blood transfusion*. Every half-hour that blood transfusion is delayed decreases the patient's chances of recovery.

What must a first aider do?

The first aider's duty is plain. It is to speed the removal of the severely injured patient to a properly equipped hospital, doing only what is necessary meanwhile to prevent the shock getting worse. If the severely injured patient is in hospital within half-an-hour, the first aider will have played a major part in saving life.

Mythology of shock

Shock is an area about which medical ideas of causes and treatment have repeatedly changed over the years. These changes have inevitably been reflected in first aid teaching. The consequence has been muddle and confusion. Now the facts are becoming clear and from the first aider's point of view, they can be stated quite simply. But first the muddle must be cleared away.

Some first aid teachers actually describe six kinds of shock:

- primary,
- secondary,
- haemorrhagic,
- traumatic,
- toxic *and*
- nervous.

(a) *Primary shock* is fainting, and the condition popularly spoken of as 'shock' following an unpleasant experience or a nasty shake-up. We shall describe it later (*see* page 59).

(b) *Secondary shock* or *established shock* is true wound shock, with which we are concerned here.

(c) *Haemorrhagic shock* is, again, true wound shock, emphasising the importance of bleeding in its cause.

(d) *Traumatic shock* is also true wound shock. The word *traumatic* is the adjective of *trauma*, which simply means 'injury'.

(e) *Toxic shock* is a rare condition, coming on four or more hours after severe injury and therefore almost never seen by the first aider at work.

(f) *Nerve shock* or *nervous shock* is a meaningless term, since there are nervous factors in every case of shock. These nervous factors range from purely psychological anxiety to the excruciating pain following a blow in the solar plexus or on the testicle.

From this point on, we shall use the word *shock* only for true wound shock, that is, for (b), (c) and (d) above.

The shocked patient

The shocked patient may display some or all of the following symptoms:

1   facial expression seems anxious, or the patient is staring in a vacant way;
2   skin-colour is pale – white, ashen-grey, or slightly blue;
3   the skin feels cold, yet in spite of this it may be soaked in sweat;
4   the patient is sometimes restless, fidgety, and even talkative, but may be dull, and sometimes even unconscious;
5   the breathing is rapid and shallow, sometimes sighing;
6   the pulse is usually rapid and feeble, though occasionally normal;
7   the patient usually complains little of pain, but may complain greatly of thirst;
8   there may be external signs of the cause of shock, such as injury or bloody vomit.

The first aider is not expected to measure the blood-pressure. In shock it is always low or even very low and the body temperature is subnormal. The first aider can feel the *carotid* pulse (in the neck) by placing the index finger just below the point of the jaw. Slowly slide the finger down the neck until a pulse is felt. Practise on yourself.

We can sum up the picture of the shocked patient thus: anxious, pale, cold, sweating, restless; shallow breathing, rapid pulse, usually little pain, much thirst. But remember that a shocked patient does not always show *all* of these things at the same time, for example, a patient with shock due to a heart attack or a bad fracture may be in great pain.

What happens in shock

Shock is due to **loss of body fluid**.

This happens in four different ways:

(a) Bleeding
(b) Loss of Plasma
(c) Vomiting
(d) Sweating

Bleeding

This may be:

(a) external, from the outer surface of the body; *or*

(b) internal, from the inner surfaces of the body into the stomach or gut, for example, from a bleeding stomach ulcer; *or*

(c) into the soft tissues of the body, for example, around the broken ends of a bone.

Plasma

Plasma is the fluid part of the blood (that is, blood minus red cells). The capillaries are the small tubes which join the arteries to the veins. They are the finest blood vessels of all and they have the thinnest walls. Those which start to leak in shock are:

(a) at the site of the injury, especially if the injury is a crush or a burn; *and*

(b) in the rest of the body, probably mainly in the muscles and the gut.

Each of these four ways of losing body fluid must be looked at in rather more detail. But here we must notice that the fluid in each case comes either directly or indirectly from the blood. Moreover, the more rapid the blood loss, the smaller is the amount needed to produce shock. By contrast, a much greater blood loss can be borne without symptoms of shock, provided it occurs sufficiently slowly.

Bleeding as a cause of shock

Actual blood loss is now regarded as by far the most important factor in producing shock after serious injury.

External blood loss can be *seen*, and as already mentioned, the blood should be mopped up and collected and sent with the patient to hospital, to help the surgeon to judge how much has been lost. If this is not possible an estimate should be made of the quantity and sent, in writing, with the patient.

Internal blood loss may be caused by injury or by bleeding from an ulcer in the stomach or bowel. In the latter case the blood may be vomited up, or passed in a motion. The condition of shock does not differ in any way at all from that produced by external bleeding.

There may be no visible external injury even though internal organs are damaged and bleeding. A careful history of the accident will indicate the possibility of internal damage and the need to watch for signs of shock.

Blood loss into the tissues themselves can be equally important as a cause of shock. If a large bone is broken, there will usually be a great deal of bleeding into the tissues around the broken ends, even though nothing shows from outside. This internal bruising can be detected by measuring the amount of swelling of a limb. A broken shinbone (or tibia) will cause an internal bleeding of about a pint of blood, not really enough on its own to produce shock. A broken thigh bone (or femur), however, will cause two-and-a-half to three pints of hidden internal bleeding, with quite considerable shock as a result.

Capillary leakage

When tissues are injured they produce certain chemical substances which pass into the blood. These substances affect specifically the capillaries in the immediate vicinity of the injury and also the capillaries throughout the body. Their general effect on the body can be shown in the following way: if the veins from the injured part are temporarily blocked, the degree of shock is reduced; and when the block is released, the shock gets worse.

The capillaries immediately affected are first caused to dilate. This means that some of the body's blood stagnates here, out of effective use. Next, the walls of the capillaries begin to leak, so that the fluid part of the blood can seep away (see Fig. 5.1). The result is a further reduction in the amount of available blood.

This seeping away of the fluid part of the blood is specially important

Normal Capillaries

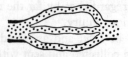

Dilated Capillaries

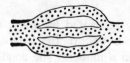

Dilated Leaking Capillaries

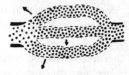

Figure 5.1   The capillaries in shock: (top) normal capillaries – the dots are the red blood cells; (middle) in shock the affected capillaries first dilate so that blood stagnates in them, thus reducing the amount of blood circulating; (bottom) the capillaries start to leak and the fluid part of the blood seeps away. The red blood cells are too large to escape through the leaks; as a result, the loss of fluid increases their concentration so that the blood becomes thicker and stickier

in extensive burns. The capillaries in the burnt area itself become very leaky indeed, and huge quantities of fluid can be lost from the burnt surface. One result of this is that the blood which remains becomes thicker and stickier. In severe burns, local fluid loss is of paramount importance in producing shock.

Apart from severe burns, capillary leakage is a major factor in producing shock whenever there is substantial damage or destruction of living tissue. Such injury is usually due to accidents, from falls, collapsing buildings, pinning under vehicles, machine injuries, in which limbs are crushed in rollers or torn off by machinery.

Vomiting and sweating

Vomiting and sweating both occur as reactions to intense anxiety or severe pain. Both tend to make shock a little worse than it otherwise would be, but by themselves they seldom involve enough fluid loss to cause serious harm.

The sweat on a cold skin, which the shocked person so often shows, may be due neither to anxiety nor to pain. The skin has become cold as a means of cutting down heat loss from the body; and sweat which would normally evaporate unnoticed remains on the skin as clammy beads of perspiration.

Pain

Painful nerve stimuli play a small part only, mainly at the start of shock. If the nerves from the injured part are blocked, the degree of shock is reduced. Despite this, however, it is doubtful if pain on its own can produce real shock; minor injuries can be excruciatingly painful, for example, a torn-off nail, and may cause fall of blood pressure or fainting but do not cause real shock.

Results of fluid loss

Once it is realised that the fundamental cause of shock is lack of blood in circulation, the other changes are easily understood. Most of them are attempts by the rest of the body to make up for this lack of blood:

- the heart works faster to get what blood there is around;
- the lungs do the same to get all the oxygen they can to the reduced amount of blood;
- the skin blood vessels contract, to cut down loss of heat from the body.

But if internal bleeding or the seeping-away of body fluid continues, the body can do nothing more to compensate. The pulse gets weaker, the breathing alternates between big sighing and little shallow movements, consciousness is clouded and then lost, and the patient finally dies because too little blood is reaching the brain.

Management of shock

It should now be clear that shock is certain to follow all severe crushes, tissue-tearing injuries, burns, major bleeding from wounds or from the stomach, and breaks of the larger bones. The mere occurrence of one of these injuries or conditions is enough to lead to the decision that the patient is suffering from shock.

Because the only life-saving treatment of shock is blood transfusion, we prefer to speak of the work of the first aider as management rather than treatment of shock. This is what a first aider must do.

1   Call an ambulance as soon as really serious injury is apparent. Also telephone the hospital to warn the casualty department that a severely injured and shocked patient is on the way.

2   Keep the patient still. The patient should be moved only if absolutely necessary, and then only enough to get him or her out of danger and made comfortable. The principle to be followed is utmost gentleness. Methods of moving the shocked or unconscious patient will be discussed later (*see* page 148).

3   Cover wounds and check external bleeding.

4   Loosen clothing, especially tight clothing round the neck, chest and waist, but no clothes should be removed.

5   Warmth. If the weather is cold, the patient should be covered with an overcoat or a blanket. In warm weather no covering is needed.

6   Remember to be calm and cheerful. The first aider should be quietly cheerful and confident. There should be no anxious over-activity or forced jollity. Remember that the shocked patient can still have an acute sense of hearing, so do not discuss a patient's condition unless well out of earshot.

We now have to consider four rather more controversial aspects of the management of shock:

- position
- heat
- fluids
- morphia.

Position

In theory, it is a good thing to raise the legs and lower the head of the shocked patient, so as to increase the blood flow to the brain. In practice, unless the patient is already on a stretcher, first aid attempts are likely to do more harm than good. If the patient is on a stretcher, the foot end may be raised nine inches, provided it can be done without risking a spill. Otherwise, leave well alone.

Do not put anything under the shocked patient's head to raise it; this is dangerous as it reduces the blood flow to the brain. The exceptions to this rule are severe injuries to the chest or stomach, when pillows or folded blankets under the head and shoulders will give added comfort and safety.

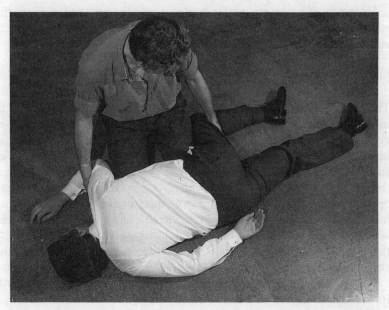

Figure 5.2   The recovery position. The patient has been rolled gently on to the side and the first aider has bent the upper arm and leg to support the patient's shoulder and hips. The lower arm is extended behind the body and the face is turned towards the ground so that saliva and vomit can run out of the mouth and the airway can be kept clear

If the patient is vomiting, or is semi-conscious or unconscious, and the injuries permit, he or she should be gently rolled into the *recovery position* (*see* Fig. 5.2). Once again, there should be nothing placed under the head to raise it.

Heat

In the past keeping the patient warm was regarded as the standard treatment of shock, and first aiders were told to use hot-water bottles and even electric cradles. But the reason why the patient feels cold is that the blood vessels in the skin have all closed down as the body attempts to force what little blood is available to the brain and other vital organs. Lack of blood in the skin does no harm. If external heat is applied, blood will be drawn away from the vital places where it is needed, and the patient will suffer.

Shocked patients who are not warmed recover as well as or even better than those who were warmed.

Moreover, if hot-water bottles or electric cradles are used, there is the additional danger of skin burns during the period when consciousness and sensitivity to pain are diminished.

Fluids

The shocked patient is often intensely thirsty; this is nature's response to blood and fluid loss. Part of the traditional treatment for shock was giving hot sweet tea, this is now realised to be a dangerous practice. As has already been emphasised, the first principle in the management of shock is to get the patient to hospital as swiftly as possible. On arrival there, the surgeon may well decide that, besides transfusion, immediate operation is essential. But the dangers of anaesthetising someone who has just been drinking any fluids, are considerable and so surgery is delayed and vital hours are lost. With stomach injuries, there is the added danger that any fluid drunk will leak out of the stomach or gut into the abdominal cavity.

It follows that the only safe rule is: **no fluids of any kind by mouth to the shocked patient**.

The same absolute prohibition applies to giving chocolate or boiled sweets to suck. If, however, the patient complains of thirst, he or she may be allowed to rinse the mouth with water and spit it out, or, better still, the lips may be moistened with a damp tissue.

Painkillers

The actual giving of strong painkillers, such as morphia, is no concern of the first aider, but it may be necessary to call the doctor so that morphia may be given. Painkillers are not a treatment for shock but a means of relieving pain. It is needed *only* if pain is continuous and severe – as, for example, when a limb is trapped in machinery. Obviously it will not be necessary if the patient is unconscious. Because it may take a doctor an hour or more to reach the site of a disaster in a coal mine, first aiders in coal mines may be given special powers under the law to administer painkillers. For this they have to be specially trained.

Other aspects of serious injuries
Crush injuries

Severe crushes, with much destruction of muscle tissue, involve an added risk besides shock. Debris and poisons from the crushed muscle released into the blood may damage or even destroy the kidneys. The resulting condition is called the *crush syndrome*. The same kind of kidney damage may follow severe burns.

Injury to the abdomen may cause damage to the internal organs, the liver, spleen or bowels. There may be internal bleeding with no external injury; patients are shocked and show signs of blood loss. The history of the injury is most important. Crush injuries of this type most commonly occur in mining and train disasters. In industry, a limb may be trapped between rollers, or part of the body may be crushed by a falling beam or masonry, or by the collapse of a trench in civil engineering operations. The patient should be released as swiftly as possible. If breathing has stopped, artificial respiration (*see* page 115) should be commenced at once. The general care of the crush injury follows precisely the same lines as for shock.

1   Call an ambulance
2   Keep the patient still
3   Cover wounds and check bleeding
4   Loosen clothing

Again, in crush injuries, as with shock from other causes, one rule for first aiders must be: **no fluids by mouth**. To the best of rules, however, there have to be occasional exceptions. When there is bound to be great delay in getting a shocked patient to hospital, either because of distance or because the patient is trapped, and when there is no abdominal injury, it is inhuman and unnecessary to refuse the shocked patient a drink if it is asked for. But water only should be given, and in half-cupfuls only at a time. A big drink taken suddenly may produce nausea and vomiting.

Fainting

At first sight, a person who has fainted looks *shocked*: there is extreme pallor, with beads of cold sweat on the forehead; it may be impossible to feel the pulse; breathing may be shallow and sighing. But in a few moments recovery starts and consciousness begins to return.

Causes
The cause of fainting may be mental – such as the sight of blood, fear of an injection, or sudden bad news – or physical, such as extreme pain, heat or standing for a long time.

The mechanism is not unlike that which causes shock. Nerve impulses from the brain allow the capillaries in the muscles and gut to dilate, and blood stagnates in these capillaries. Lack of blood supply to the brain produces first giddiness, pallor and yawning, then unconsciousness. As a rule, the circumstances in which fainting occurs make the diagnosis obvious.

Treatment
The only treatment needed is to loosen any tight clothing around the neck; if consciousness does not return within two minutes, the patient should be rolled into the *recovery position* (*see* Fig. 5.2) and expert help sent for, as there may be some more serious cause for the unconsciousness.

The patient who feels about to faint can usually prevent this by pulling the stomach, buttock and leg muscles tight, and holding them tight a minute or so.

Review questions

1   What is *true shock*? What are the symptoms and what can the first aider do?
2   How would you distinguish an ordinary faint from other causes of unconsciousness? What would you do?

Also try the questions on severe injury on page 164.

6 Strains, sprains and fractures

Strains and sprains

A *strain* is an injury to a muscle or tendon. A *sprain* is an injury to a joint. With both strains and sprains, the first aider's prime duty is to make sure that other and more serious injury is not being passed by undetected. Often the decision will be beyond the first aider; indeed, even the most experienced expert may need an x-ray to make sure. It follows that, if there is the least doubt, the patient should be referred to a trained nurse or doctor.

Strains

The story of a strain is usually characteristic. Sharp pain in a muscle or tendon follows a sudden, energetic movement. The affected part is held stiff. The muscles most commonly strained are those of the back.

A severe strain may involve the complete rupture of a muscle or tendon. The pain is more severe, there may be great swelling, and the affected part cannot be moved. Such cases will probably need surgical treatment.

A simple strain need not be rested; active movement from the start hastens recovery. To relieve pain, a cold compress or an ice pack may be applied. Treatment with an infra-red lamp is sometimes helpful; though such treatment is outside the scope of first aid, it is often available in medical departments or industrial health centres.

Many industrial strains, particularly those of the back, can and should be prevented by modern mechanical handling methods. When manual labour cannot be avoided, proper techniques should be learnt; the motive power should come from the hip and thigh muscles, bending at the hips and knees, rather than from the back muscles, bending at the spine (*see* Fig. 6.1). There is, too, a right and a wrong way to carry heavy objects (*see* Fig. 6.2).

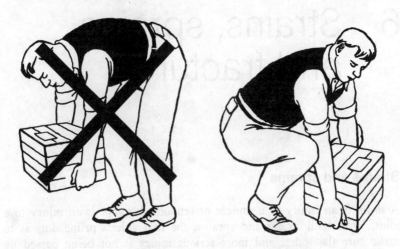

Figure 6.1   Lifting a heavy weight: (left) the wrong way is to use the muscles of the back – under great strain these muscles may tear or a weak spinal disc may slip. The feet are together, the knees are straight and the back is bent; (right) the correct way is to use the muscles to the hips and thighs. The feet are apart, the knees are bent and the back is straight

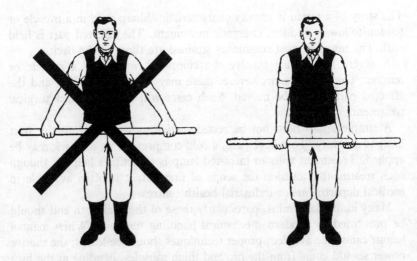

Figure 6.2   Holding an iron bar: (left) the wrong way, with the arms at right angles to the chest and both hands on the same side of the bar, placing unnecessary strain on the comparatively weak shoulder joints and on the fingers – the bar can easily slip and injure the feet; (right) the right way involves a minimum of physical effort and reduces the chances of the bar slipping

Sprains

Sprains are produced by the same kinds of injury which produce fractures. Indeed both are often present, and it is only possible to make sure no bones are broken by taking an x-ray picture.

In a sprain, the ligaments and other soft parts around the joint are either stretched or actually torn. The story is usually of either a twist or a wrench. There is pain at the point of injury and the joint is held stiff. Swelling may be considerable.

Among the commonest sprains are the footballer's sprained knee and the sprained external ligaments of the ankle. Like strains, sprains are best not rested but moved actively from the start. A cold compress will relieve pain. Cotton wool and a firm bandage will give comfort; this is the best first aid treatment.

If the pain in leg injuries is bearable, boots should be left on to make good splints; the laces, however, should be loosened. If pain is very severe, the cause is usually pressure from the swelling; the boot must then be removed. Once the boot is taken off, it will be hard, if not impossible, to get it back on again.

Dislocations

A dislocation is the displacement of one or more bones at a joint. Dislocations are much less common than either fractures or sprains.

There is loss of movement in the dislocated joint and the joint looks peculiar. The pain is often described as *sickening*. Often the patient can tell what has happened. With some joints it may have happened before.

The joint most commonly dislocated is the shoulder, usually following a fall on the outstretched hand; next, the jaw, usually following a big yawn; next, the ankle, usually with a fracture as well. Thumb and finger joints are sometimes dislocated. It needs great violence to dislocate either the elbow or the knee.

The first aid treatment is to support the part beyond the dislocation in the position of greatest comfort and to get expert help. The first aider must never try to put back a dislocation, as this may cause a fracture.

Quite often, a dislocation and a fracture occur together. Diagnosis of these double injuries is beyond the first aider, and, again, it may be impossible without an x-ray. First aid treatment is to support the part in the position of greatest comfort, and to get expert help.

Fractures

A *fracture* is a broken or cracked bone. Fractures are common in street and riding accidents; in industrial accidents they are comparatively rare. In our experience, the bones most often broken in industry are the small bones of the hands and feet, usually as a result of objects falling. The value of specially-strengthened protective boots as a means of preventing fractures, especially for workers in heavier industry and the building trades, cannot be too strongly stressed. Conversely, boots or shoes with rubber or canvas uppers are a real source of danger to the worker.

First aid care of fractures

In industry, because skilled help can almost always be quickly obtained, the first aider's role in fracture treatment is confined to true first aid. The transport of a patient with a fracture of the thigh, for example, is a task for the skilled and experienced ambulance worker, who is handling such cases every week. Usually the first aider's role is to look after the patient until the expert arrives. But with a suspected fracture of the arm, hand or foot, the first aider may well have to get the patient ready for transport as an out patient to the hospital or industrial health centre.

Serious fractures
The *seriously injured* patient will often have one or more fractures. Here treatment of the patient's general condition must have priority; care of the fracture will be limited to making the part as comfortable as possible.

With the patient who has sustained a *moderate and local injury*, the first aider must always remember the possibility of a fracture. In such cases, help should be sent for or the patient should be referred to the medical department, health centre or hospital. If there is any reason at all to suspect a fracture, the first aider must follow treatment advised to make sure that it gets no worse (*see* page 72).

Transport of severe fractures takes special training and practice. The ambulance worker must know all this, and so must a first aid worker in a coal-mine. The first aider at work, as we shall see, needs to know only certain basic principles and how to apply them if the need arises (*see* page 73).

Types of fracture

There are many varieties of fracture but for the first aider at work, only two are important – *closed* or *simple*; and *open* or *compound*. Most fractures are closed. Open fractures are so rare that many first aiders will never see one.

An open or compound fracture is one where there is an outside wound as well as a fracture, and a communication between the skin and air and the broken bone ends. This greatly increases the risk of germs getting into bones. The first aider can tell a compound fracture if there is a broken bone end sticking out from a wound or through the skin, or if broken bone is visible in a wound. But in most compound fractures, the bone cannot be seen in the wound. The best the first aider can do is to say there is a wound outside and a broken bone inside; whether they communicate is a matter for the surgeon.

The safe rule is to treat the injury as a wound – that is to say, cover it as quickly as possible with a large individual sterilised dressing in order to keep out any further infection. Once this is done, the patient's general condition and the fracture itself can be attended to. It is particularly important to handle any such injury extremely gently. One rough move-ment may link together an outside wound and an inside fracture and so convert a closed into an open fracture.

Is there a fracture?

For the first aider there are only two certain signs of a fracture:

1 If conscious, the patient may say that he or she heard or felt a bone snap.
2 The limb or injured part is often bent in a way which could happen only if the bone was broken. This is called the *deformity*; it can usually be detected without removing the clothes. Deformity is best appreciated by comparing the injured and uninjured limbs.

Everything else must be suspicion only. With many fractures, including many of those of the fingers and toes, wrist and ankle, pain is the only indication of trouble and diagnosis is impossible without an x-ray. The only safe course is for every injury with pain over or near a bone to be seen by a trained nurse or doctor.

Fractures of individual bones

Here we are concerned with bones other than the spine which will be considered later (*see* page 76). Certain bones are particularly liable to get broken. In discussing each, pictures speak louder than words. Each illustration here should be studied carefully as the text is read. In particular, attention should be paid to the way the displacement of the broken bones produces changes in the outside shape of the part of the body affected.

Collar bone or clavicle

Look at Fig. 6.3. The cause is usually a fall on the outstretched hand. The arm is held tight against the side of the chest, and any movement gives pain over the collar bone.

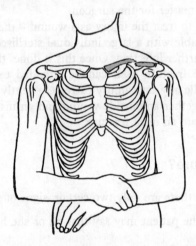

Figure 6.3   Broken collar bone or clavicle. Note that the broken ends of the bone overlap slightly, that the back of the head is turned and tilted towards the injured side, that the arm is held against the side of the chest and the forearm is supported by the other hand

Upper arm bone or humerus

Look at Fig. 6.4. Again the arm is held tight against the side of the chest, but this time pain on movement is over the broken humerus.

Forearm bones: the radius and ulna

Look at Fig. 6.5. The injured forearm is supported with the other hand. There will be pain at the site of the break. The amount of deformity depends on the extent of the breaking. A young person may crack one of the forearm bones only part of the way through; this is called a *green-stick fracture*. If one bone alone is broken, the other will act as a splint.

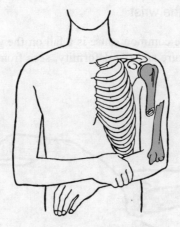

Figure 6.4 Broken humerus. As with the broken collar bone, the arm is held to the side and the forearm supported by the other hand. The broken bone ends overlap slightly so, compared with the good side, the upper arm appears to be shorter

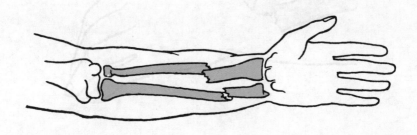

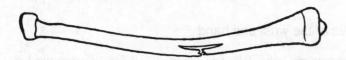

Figure 6.5 Broken radius and ulna: (top) complete break of both bones; (bottom) partial break of the radius without separation of the broken bone ends, the so called *green stick* fracture

Forearm bones at the wrist

Look at Fig. 6.6. The common cause is a fall on the wrist. The fracture is called Colles's fracture and the deformity, seen from the side, is like a dinner fork.

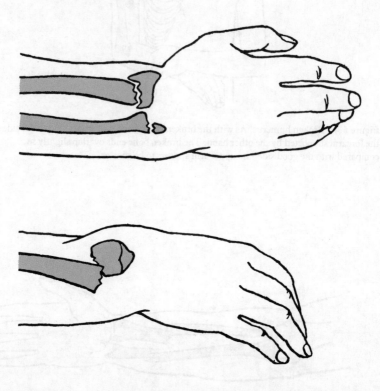

Figure 6.6   Broken wrist: (top) from the back the wrist merely looks swollen; (bottom) the break is really of the forearm bones just above the wrist. Note that the 'dinnerfork' deformity is seen only in side view. For simplicity, only one bone, the ulna, is shown

Small bones of the wrist and hand

The usual causes are jerks, falls and blows. *Chauffeurs' fracture* used to follow a backfire while using a starting handle; though now rare with cars, it still occurs with diesel engines.

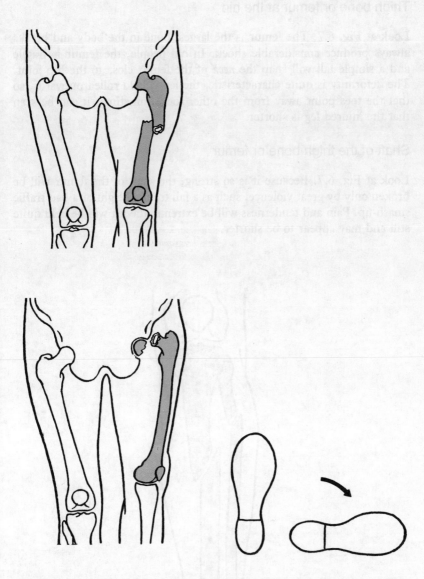

Figure 6.7 Broken thigh: (top) broken shaft of the thigh bone or femur. Note that the bone ends overlap so that the leg is shortened; but the foot is not turned out, as with a broken hip; (bottom) broken thigh bone or femur at the hip. Though usually spoken of as a broken hip the injury is really a break of the narrow neck of the femur. The main shaft of the femur is pulled up by the powerful thigh muscles, so the injured leg is made to appear shorter; (inset) position of feet with a 'broken hip' – the toes of the injured side point outwards in stead of forwards

Thigh bone or femur at the hip

Look at Fig. 6.7. The femur is the largest bone in the body and breaks always produce considerable shock. In old people, the femur is fragile and a simple fall will snap the *neck* of the femur close to the hip joint. The deformity is quite characteristic: the leg is held rolled outwards, so that the toes point away from the other foot. Sometimes it can be seen that the injured leg is shorter.

Shaft of the thigh bone or femur

Look at Fig. 6.7. Because it is so strong, the shaft of the femur will be broken only by great violence, such as a fall from a height or a bad traffic smash-up. Pain and tenderness will be extreme; the leg will be held quite still and may appear to be shorter.

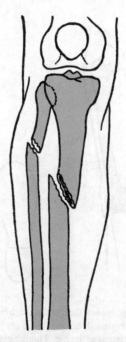

Figure 6.8   Broken shin bones. The large shin bone, the tibia, lies just under the skin so the break may be felt by running the finger down the bone. A break of the small shinbone, the fibula, cannot be detected in this way. If both bones are broken the ends overlap so the leg is shortened

Shin bones: the tibia and fibula

Look at Fig. 6.8. The large shin bone, the tibia, is just under the skin, so a break can be felt quite easily by running a finger along it. As a rule, the thin little fibula is broken as well. The common causes are football injuries, road accidents and falls.

Shin bones at the ankle

Look at Fig. 6.9. It is usually impossible for the first aider to distinguish a badly strained ankle from a broken one. The cause is usually a twist or a fall, often a slight one. Sometimes the whole foot is pushed backwards on the leg, the characteristic deformity of *Potts's fracture* in which, besides the broken bones, the ankle is dislocated.

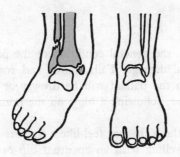

Figure 6.9   Broken ankle. The break is really of the shin bones just above and at the side of the ankle. The swelling is usually so great that the break can be detected only by x-ray examination

Small bones of the ankle and foot

The possibility of fracture should be borne in mind whenever a weight is dropped on the foot or toe.

Ribs

Look at Fig. 6.10. Rib fractures are common. They may be caused by sudden compression of the chest, or by falls, for example, on the corner of a workbench. There is usually no deformity, but there may be sharp pain on breathing or coughing.

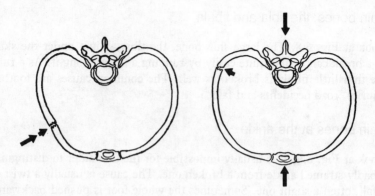

Figure 6.10 Broken rib: diagrammatic sectional view. Arrows show the direction of forces producing injuries. The break is produced (left) by direct force, (right) by compression of chest

Skull

With head injuries, the general condition of the patient matters much more than the local damage. Falls, blows and road accidents are the usual causes. Often the patient will be drowsy or unconscious. Blood from the nose or ear, following a blow on the head, suggests a broken skull.

A bad bruise on the scalp may feel like a fracture of the skull; there is a raised circular swelling with an apparent dip or hole in the centre. Usually there is no break, but this is a matter for a trained nurse or a doctor to decide.

Care of fractures

The principle of first aid care of any fracture is to steady the broken bone ends so that the patient can move or be moved without added pain or further injury. Remember the following points.

1 Keep the injured part still. The injured part should be steadied and supported to prevent movement of the broken bone ends. With long bones, this means that the joints at each end of the broken bone must be held still.

2 Do not use force. If the limb is in a very unnatural position, it should be moved with great care and without force into as natural a position as possible. If it is not in a very unnatural position, it should not be moved.

3   Fix the injured part in a natural position. If the patient is to move, or to be moved, without further expert help, the injured part should be fixed in a comfortable natural position. Fixing is done with triangular bandages, opened out or folded, plenty of cotton wool padding, and with the body, another limb, or a piece of wood used as a splint.

4   Do not move clothing. Do not try to remove the patient's clothes; this may do further damage by moving the broken bone-ends.

Immobilising or fixing of hip, thigh and shin fractures

Patients with fractures of the hip, thigh and shin will normally be transported to hospital by ambulance as quickly as possible. Any splinting needed will therefore usually be done by the expert ambulance men.

If, for any reason, the first aider does have to splint a fractured hip, thigh or shin, the safest way is to tie the two limbs together with four to six folded triangular bandages. An assistant may at the same time exert a steady pull on the foot, without bending or turning it in any way. This pull is to overcome, or at least reduce, the muscle spasm around the fracture, which is the main cause of the pain (*see* Fig. 6.11).

Plenty of cotton wool should be placed round the injured limb before the two bandages are applied *on either side* of the fracture. *Never* bandage directly over a fracture.

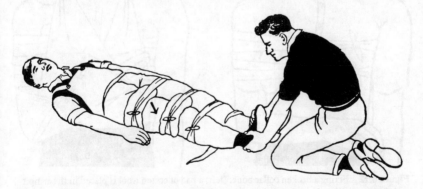

Figure 6.11   Splinting a broken hip, thigh or shin. For simplicity, the first aider doing the bandaging is not shown. The arrow indicates the position of the suspected break. An assistant exerts a steady pull on the foot, without bending or turning it while the bad leg is tied to the good leg with folded triangular bandages. Plenty of cotton wool is placed round the injured limb before the two bandages are applied just above and below the fracture

As we have seen, on no account should any attempt be made to remove the clothes. It is reasonable, however, to roll up the trouser or pull down the stocking to see if a fractured shin bone has penetrated the skin.

Once the limb is properly immobilised, the patient may be lifted carefully on to a stretcher.

Other fractures

Patients with severe head injuries will go straight to hospital under expert care; they will usually be unconscious and the fractured skull needs no first aid. Details will be given later when the unconscious patient is considered (*see* page 102).

Unless they are shocked, patients with fractures or suspected fractures of the arm and forearm, wrist and ankle, hand and foot, collar bone and ribs can be moved to the medical department, health centre, or hospital by car as sitting patients. For such patients, then, first aid fixing may be necessary.

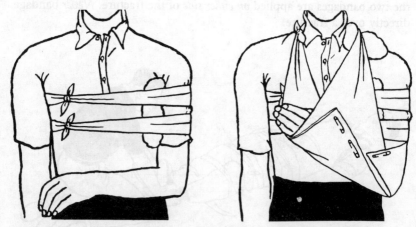

Figure 6.12 Fixing a broken collar bone: (left) a pad of cotton wool is placed in the armpit and the upper arm is bound to the side of the chest by two folded triangular bandages; (right) the forearm is supported in a sling at an angle of 45 degrees and a large cotton wool pad is placed between the sling and the injured shoulder. Alternatively, a clove hitch (*see* Fig. 2.7) may be used or, for those who have learnt its use, the special St John sling. The object of the first method is to lever out gently the point of the shoulder. The object of the second is to take the weight of the arm off the injured bone

Fixing of other individual fractures

With suspected fractures around the shoulder or in the arm or forearm, it is usually enough to apply carefully and gently an ordinary right-angle sling, without removing the clothing. The conventional methods of splinting are illustrated below. Look carefully at each drawing and read the treatment described in the caption.

Ankle
Pad all round with cotton wool, and bandage firmly. No weight should be borne on the injured ankle.

Hands and feet
Fractures of the small bones of the hand and foot, fingers and toes require no first aid splinting. The injured hand should be rested in a sling. No weight should be borne on the injured foot.

Ribs
Fractures of the ribs require no first aid splinting. If pain is extreme, this may be eased by propping up with several pillows.

Using bandages and slings
Whenever bandages or slings are used for fixing fractures, these must be secured firmly enough but not too tight. Too tight a bandage will cause the part below it to start to swell.

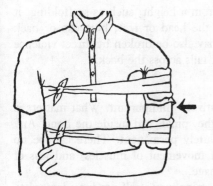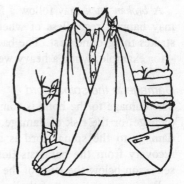

Figure 6.13 Fixing a broken humerus: (left) the side of the chest is used as a splint. A large pad of cotton wool is placed between the arm and the chest, and cotton wool is placed round the arm above and below the break. The arm is bound to the chest with two folded triangular bandages; (right) the forearm is supported in a sling at a right angle

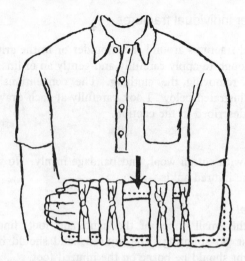

Figure 6.14   Fixing a broken radius and ulna. A simple splint padded with cotton wool extends from the elbow to the knuckles along the palm surface of the forearm and hand. Note the cotton wool pads under the bandages on each side of the fracture. The forearm is carried in a right angle sling

Fractured spine

The spine may be broken in the neck or the back. A *broken neck* may follow a fall on to the head or the sudden stop when a car, motor-cycle, plane or train crashes. The head jerks forward or backwards, and snaps the neck.

A *broken back* may follow a fall from a height, such as scaffolding; it may happen regardless of whether the head or feet, buttocks or back strikes the ground first. The back may also be broken by direct violence – for example, when a heavy weight falls across the back.

Damage to the spinal cord
The damage to the bone is comparatively unimportant. What matters is damage, or the risk of damage, to the spinal cord inside the bone. Any damage to the spinal cord is absolutely permanent. There can be no recovery from the paralysis (loss of movement of muscles) and loss of sensation below the level of the damage.

Because movement of the broken spine may itself produce damage to the spinal cord, the first aider should if avoidable, do *absolutely nothing*.

The first aider will suspect or recognise a broken spine by the following:

(a) the story of the accident;
(b) pain at the place of injury;
(c) the patient feels 'afraid to move' or may be unable to move.

If it is absolutely necessary to move the patient or adjust his position, it must be done very gently and slowly. The greatest care must be taken not to bend up the back or neck or twist the spine. How *not* to do it is shown in Fig. 6.15.

For anything more than the slightest movement, head and foot traction should be used, preferably with four people helping (*see* Fig. 6.16). But it must be emphasised that this is a job for expert first aiders who have practised the manoeuvre carefully.

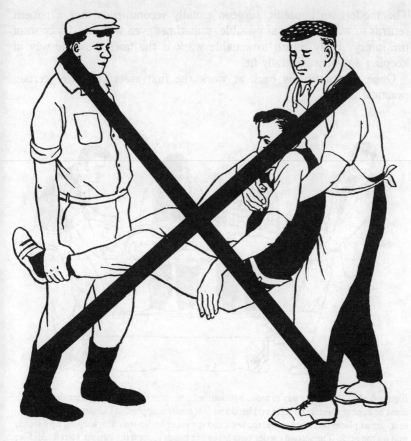

Figure 6.15   The *wrong* way to move a patient with an injured back. It is called *jack-knifing*. If the spine is injured it is certain to cause damage to the spinal cord

If lifting is absolutely necessary, then the opportunity should be taken to put the patient on to a flat hard stretcher without pillows, or on to a door. But the proper course is always to wait for the expert *ambulance men*, unless there is an overwhelming reason for not doing so.

If the patient with a broken back is found lying on his face, he may with advantage be transported on his or her front.

With a broken neck, the patient should be moved on his or her back, with the head supported between two rolled blankets, sand-bags, or bricks wrapped in cotton wool.

The recovering fracture

The modern orthopaedic surgeon usually recommends that a patient returns to work as soon as possible, sometimes even within a day or so of the injury. Early return to suitable work is the finest possible way of keeping a patient generally fit.

Once the patient is back at work the first aider can offer certain practical advice.

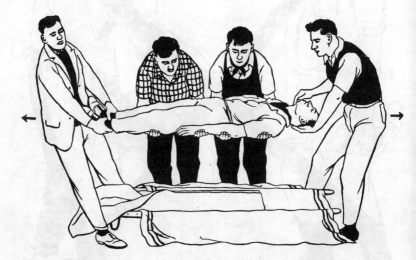

Figure 6.16   The *correct* way to move a patient with an injured back. The patient's spine must be kept absolutely straight and head and foot traction applied at the same time. The first carrier places one hand under the neck and the other under the chin, keeping up a steady pull on the neck. The second carrier puts his or her hands around the patient's heels. All four carriers must move very slowly and carefully and in complete unison. It is best, however, not to move the patient at all, but to wait for expert ambulance help

- A plaster splint should not be covered with a rubber glove; the retained sweat softens the plaster.
- Avoid rubbing a plaster or getting suds or water on it.
- The patient with crutches or in plaster must be encouraged to move around from time to time and not remain sitting in one place.
- The rubbers on the ends of crutches must be in good repair.

Review questions

1   What are the signs of a fractured bone? What is the general aim of first aid treatment to a fracture?
2   How would you treat an old lady who had fallen onto her left side and complained of pain in her hip?

Also try the questions on fractures on page 164.
Also try the questions on fractures on page 164.

7 Burns and scalds, electrical and heat injuries

Burns

A *burn* is tissue damage produced by *dry* heat; a *scald* is damage by *wet* heat. Tissue damage produced by the direct action of a strong chemical is referred to as a *chemical burn*.

The seriousness of any burn depends on four factors:

(a) area;
(b) depth;
(c) part of body affected; *and*
(d) the age of the patient.

Area of burn

The skin *area* involved in a burn is more important than the *depth*. In estimating the extent of the burnt *area*, the *rule of nines* will be found helpful. The body surface divides up conveniently and sufficiently accurately for first aid purposes into the following *percentage* areas:

Area	Percentage
Each arm	9
Head and neck	9
Each leg	18
Front of trunk	18
Back of trunk	18

Even a superficial burn involving more than five per cent of the body surface is serious; if more than fifteen per cent of the surface is involved, the condition is extremely dangerous, and the patient may die of shock, unless blood transfusion is started within an hour or so.

In all large burns, there is severe shock, due to the great quantities of fluid lost both from the raw surface and into the damaged tissues, as shown by the swelling of the burnt part. Naturally, the larger the burnt area, the greater the shock.

Burning sterilises the tissues, but the damage and the exposure of a large raw area greatly increase the chances of subsequent infection. The greater the area, the greater the infection risk. Good first aid will help to keep the burn clean and infection-free; bad first aid may itself introduce infection.

Depth of burn

For practical purposes two *depths* of burn have to be recognised.

Superficial burns
Only the outer layers of the skin are affected. The burnt area goes red, and blisters may or may not form. Pain is considerable, but the burn usually heals rapidly; as a rule there is little scarring. Large superficial burns produce considerable shock.

Deep burns
All the layers of the skin are damaged, and the fat and muscle beneath the skin, and even the bone, may be involved. The burnt area is yellowy-white, or actually charred. If the skin is completely destroyed, there will be less pain than in superficial burns, because the sensitive nerve endings in the skin will also have been destroyed. Deep burns often become infected. They heal very slowly, and scarring is often serious.

Part of body

Burns of the face and hands are more serious than burns of corresponding size elsewhere because quite small scarring may upset both function and appearance.

Age of patient

Children and old people react badly to severe burns. Moreover, they are particularly liable to extensive accidental burns.

Varieties of burn

Dry heat burns
These may be caused by contact with hot metal – for example, a

soldering iron or an unprotected hot-water bottle. The burn is sharply localised and may be superficial or deep.

Dry cold burns
These may be caused by contact with liquid gases, for example liquid oxygen or carbon dioxide. The burned area is sharply localised and pale.

Fire burns
These may follow a blow back from a boiler, or involvement in flaming petrol or other solvent, or a burning building; the clothes usually catch fire. Such a burn often covers a large area; parts of it may be superficial and other parts deep. Charred clothing may be stuck to the burn. The patient is usually very shocked.

Sunburn
This may follow exposure to natural or artificial sunlight. It is very superficial but there is often considerable reddening and blistering.

Friction burn
This is a rare type of burn. It is caused through catching hold of a rapidly moving rope – for example, a haulage rope in a mine.

Wet burns or scalds
These may be caused by steam, hot water, hot oils, fats (for example cooking fat), hot solvents or tar. They are usually superficial but are often extensive and therefore serious.

Radiation burn
Ionising radiations from x-rays, or radioactive materials of any kind, damage living tissues and, if sufficiently strong, can actually burn the skin. Such burn can take a very long time to heal and need specialist treatment. Skin cancer is liable to develop later on. Burns like these should never occur if the proper safety rules laid down by regulation are followed. The severe *flash burns* that occurred after the atomic explosion at Hiroshima were due to the intense heat of the explosion.

Microwave burn
High frequency radiation penetrates the skin and heats up the underlying tissues. Excessive exposure can cause a burn-like reaction under the skin which may break down in a day or two producing a deep ulcer. There will be deep pain and swelling, developing after the exposure. Medical advice must be obtained as soon as possible.

Electrical and chemical burns will be considered later (*see* pages 85 and 93).

First aid treatment of burns

In treating a burn or scald the objectives are to:

- prevent shock,
- avoid infection, and
- relieve pain.

Do not:

- allow anything bacteriologically 'dirty' to be put on the burn – such as old grease or ointment,
- touch the burn during treatment,
- speak or breathe on to the burn until the injured part is covered with a clean or sterile dressing.

For treatment purposes, burns are divided into:

(a) trivial,
(b) medium, *and*
(c) serious.

The first aider can safely treat the trivial burn, but any medium burn, that is to say, one larger than a 5p piece or an average cigarette burn, ought to receive expert treatment from a trained nurse or a doctor, so that the chances of infection may be kept to a minimum. The patient with a serious burn, involving more than a few square inches of skin, will be sent direct to hospital.

Trivial burns

Trivial burns are often very painful but can be treated effectively by remembering these points.

(a) The pain is quickly relieved by holding the burned part under running cold water.

(b) If there is any sign of injury to the skin, the burn should be carefully cleaned with hibitane, cetrimide or soap and water, and cotton wool, in the same way that minor wounds are dealt with.

(c) After cleaning, the burn and surrounding skin should be dried with clean cotton wool, and covered with an individual sterilised dressing. A better dressing to relieve pain is the sterilised *tulle gras* dressing which is contained between two slips of transparent paper. One slip is pulled off, and the dressing, still attached to the other slip, is applied. The second slip is then quite easily removed leaving the sterilised tulle gras in place. In applying the tulle gras the first aider must take care not to touch the dressing, except at the corners or edges; in separating it from the slip of paper, forceps will be helpful (*see* Fig. 7.1). If the tulle gras is too large it should be cut to the right size before the slips of paper are removed. The tulle gras is covered with a small individual sterilised dressing, an individual plaster, or clean cotton wool and a roller bandage.

(d) If there is a blister, it should not be pricked, and the first aider should not try to remove dead skin (*see* page 48).

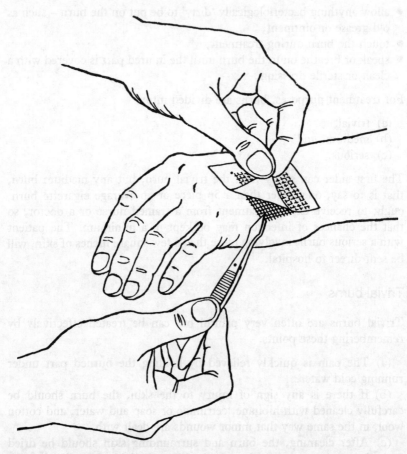

Figure 7.1 Applying tulle gras dressing to a minor burn. The dressing is held in place at one corner with forceps, while the slip of greaseproof paper is pulled off with the free hand

Medium burns

First apply cold water to the burn. Since thorough cleansing of the burnt area will be undertaken by the doctor or nurse, the first aider's next duty is simply to cover the burn with one or more individual sterilised dressings, and to get the patient to the expert as quickly as possible. There is no point in putting tulle gras on any burn which is to be efficiently cleaned within an hour or so; any oil or grease applied by the first aider simply makes the cleaning more difficult.

Serious burns

Again, first apply cold water. Remember that the burning itself will have sterilised the whole area, so *do not*:

- attempt to clean the burn;
- attempt to remove clothes or pull away charred clothing which has stuck to the burn.

The burnt area must be quickly covered with one or more large sterilised individual dressings. If the area burnt is too extensive even for this, a clean towel or sheet may be used as a covering. At hospital, cleaning will be undertaken with full surgical precautions in an operating theatre.

Rapid replacement of body fluid lost is the life-saving treatment in such cases, so rapid transport to hospital is vital. As a rule, attempts to carry out blood transfusion or even intravenous saline infusion outside hospital do more harm than good by delaying full-scale controlled fluid replacement. They are now resorted to only when the patient is trapped and cannot be quickly released, or where the journey to hospital will probably take a long time.

The general treatment of shock, as set out earlier, must be followed (*see* page 55). If the patient is thirsty, he or she may rinse out the mouth and spit out. Only if there is likely to be considerable delay in getting the patient to hospital may water, drunk in small sips only, be permitted; larger quantities of fluid taken suddenly may cause vomiting. With small burns, hot sweet tea is harmless and comforting, and may be given.

Electric burns

Causes

Electricity may cause burns, *electric shock*, or both. Burns occur at the points of entry of an electric current, that is, the points of contact with a live conductor. A common cause is worn electric cable of a portable hand tool, such as a soldering iron or drill, especially if there is inadequate earthing. A much more severe burn with extensive charring of the tissues will follow contact with a high-tension supply. Indeed, the heat and destruction from a high-tension contact are so great that the path of conduction is broken and clothes catch fire.

Symptoms

A mild electric current may produce a pattern on the skin like the branches of a tree or the meshes of wire netting. This is probably because the electricity flows along the trickles of sweat on the skin. A moderate current will produce a dry, shrivelled burn with little pain – less than from a heat burn of the same size. There is little or no reddening around the burn, and the burnt tissue takes the form of a cone with the point inwards, extending down from the skin into the deeper structures. Quite a small burn may involve tendons and other important structures, and this may not be apparent for three or four days.

Sometimes, as well as the burn at the point of entry of an electric current, there may be a similar burn at the point of exit. For example, where the entry burn is on the hand, there may be an exit burn on the foot.

Treatment

Even the smallest electric burn should be covered with a clean dry dressing and referred to a nurse or doctor. The *devitalisation* of the tissue around the burn will delay healing and increase the risk of infection. The best treatment may often prove to be a small skin-graft, usually applied in the out-patient department.

Electric shock

Electric shock is the general bodily reaction to the passage of an electric current. It may vary from slight tingling to sudden unconsciousness in which the patient may appear to be dead. But the first aider must never presume death in electric shock, for the breathing may stop and the pulse vanish, yet life can still be restored.

Direct and alternating currents
Direct current is said to be less dangerous than alternating current, for

the following reason. Direct current produces a single violent muscular contraction, which tends to throw the patient away from the source of the shock. Indeed, the resulting fall is as likely to cause injury as the shock itself. By contrast, alternating current produces continuous muscle spasm, which may cause the affected muscles of the arm and hand to grip involuntarily the source of electric supply. So a continuous prolonged shock is more likely. For this reason, an electrician who is unwise enough to test a source of alternating current by touch will do so with the back of his hand!

Low voltages
Voltages under 150–250 are not often fatal, and occasionally 800 volts have been survived. The lowest fatal voltage ever recorded was 38. A great deal depends on the contact between the source of electricity and the skin, and between the skin and the ground. If the skin, clothes or shoes are wet or moist, the shock is correspondingly greater and its effects correspondingly worse. A metal floor will also increase conductivity. A person who is fatigued stands shock worse than one who is fresh.

High voltages
With very high voltages, the current usually does not penetrate the body deeply, because the electrical pressure is so great that the tissues and conductors are destroyed.

Domestic voltages
Ordinary domestic AC current alternates at 50 cycles per second. Such a current can just be felt if it is of one milliamp. By contrast, a DC current has to reach five milliamps before it is perceptible. One hundred milliamps AC is the usual minimum fatal current, but as low a figure as 20 milliamps AC has caused death. The length of duration of exposure to a current is very important; with exposures of over five seconds, the danger of serious injury is great.

Effects of electric shock

The skin has a very high electrical resistance, about 3,000 ohms if dry and healthy. Once this resistance is overcome, the current follows the internal water courses of the body. A current passing from leg to leg does less harm than one passing from arm to leg, since the latter will pass over and often damage the electrical mechanism of the heart. A current passing from head to leg will travel via the fluid around the brain and spinal cord, damaging vital electric control centres on its way.

Most electric shocks occur among works and maintenance engineers. A third of all fatal electrical accidents are due to portable electrical apparatus and hand-tools.

A severe electric shock may occur during electric welding, where a sweaty worker is lying in contact with a metal sheet which may become live. A fatal shock may be caused by a jib-crane fouling an overhead cable; or a metal strip may touch the 'live' overhead wires feeding an electric gantry.

Symptoms

These may vary from muscle spasm and pain to unconsciousness and even deep coma. Pain in the affected muscles may be intense. Inasmuch as the patient cannot overcome the spasm of the muscles by an effort of will, the muscles are effectively paralysed, as long as the shock continues.

If it is strong enough, the electric current may paralyse the breathing muscles, or put the breathing control centre in the brain out of action. It cannot be too strongly emphasised that such a paralysis is usually transitory. At the same time, the electric current may partially paralyse the heart muscle. As a result, the heart beats rapidly but feebly, in a state of 'flutter'; in this state, although the blood is still circulating, the pulse cannot be detected. It follows that absence of both pulse and respiration in a patient unconscious from electric shock are *not* signs of death. Prolonged artificial respiration may yet save life.

Treatment

Speed and coolness are essential, and may be life-saving. The first move is to disconnect the patient from the source of the electricity:

1 Switch off the current. All first aiders should know the location of electric switches in the area of the workplace for which they are responsible.
2 If this is impossible, pull or push the patient away from the source of the electricity, while taking great care not to make electrical contact with either the ground or the patient:

(a) Stand or kneel on a dry non-conductor, such as a dry rug, mackintosh or rubber mat.
(b) Pull or push the patient away from the source of the electricity, again using a dry non-conductor. Considerable force may be needed to

get the patient free. If the patient has to be grasped, use special heavy rubber gloves, or dry sacking, a dry coat or several thicknesses of dry paper. Domestic rubber gloves give no protection against high voltages. If a crooked stick is available, this may be used, but not an umbrella, since it has metal ribs. Dry rope is another good non-conductor.

(c) Avoid contact with any part of the patient which may be moist, for example the arm-pits or crutch, or the face, which may be wet with spittle.

With very high voltages – for example, at electricity stations or in overhead wires – the patient will usually have been thrown clear. If not, the danger to a rescuer while the current is still on is very great, and all possible precautions must be taken. Remember to: **switch off the current before rescue is attempted**.

Artificial respiration

Once the patient has been rescued from contact with the electric source, if breathing has ceased or is very feeble, artificial respiration should be started at once, using the methods described later (*see* page 115). At the same time, the standard treatment for shock in an unconscious patient should be applied (*see* page 56), but this definitely takes second place to artificial respiration. Since artificial respiration may have to continue for half an hour or more, a resuscitator is of the greatest value.

In about half of all electrocution cases with cessation of breathing there is recovery with artificial respiration; nine out of ten patients who start breathing again do so within half-an-hour of artificial respiration being started. There is no record of recovery after electrocution where artificial respiration has had to continue for more than an hour. But carry on! Yours may be the first case.

Delay in starting artificial respiration can prove disastrous. If it is started *at once*, 70 per cent of the patients recover. If there is more than three minutes' delay, only 20 per cent recover. The lesson here is obvious.

Heat injuries

True *heat stroke* is a rare and somewhat dangerous condition which occurs when the overheated patient has neglected treatment and remained for some time in a very hot environment. The first, and much more common, effect of too much heat is *heat exhaustion*. This is also known as miners' or stokers' cramp.

Cause

The essential cause is loss of too much body water and body salt as a result of too little replacement to make good what has been lost by sweating. Sweating is part of the natural mechanism of cooling the body. It is not the production of sweat, but its evaporation from the body surface which uses up body heat and so lowers the body temperature. If the body is getting too little water and salt to replace what is lost as sweat, or if the surrounding air is so full of water-vapour that the sweat cannot evaporate, the body cuts down on further sweating, and the internal temperature starts to rise. If this is allowed to continue, true heat stroke develops.

Symptoms

- *Heat exhaustion*: The skin is clammy, and the patient irritable and complains of severe cramps in the limbs.
- *Early heat stroke*. The skin is hot and dry, and the irritability and cramps are much more severe.
- *Second stage of heat stroke*. The patient may be found unconscious, breathing hard and sometimes twitching a little. The skin is dry, red and burning hot.

Prevention

Among those specially liable to heat exhaustion and heat stroke are steel workers and miners. So workers at furnaces and in foundries, glass works and other very hot places should be provided with special drinks which may be flavoured with orange or lemon and glucose and may contain salt. Medical advice should be sought as too much salt can be harmful.

Working in airtight plastic protective clothing may produce heat exhaustion and heat stroke, especially if the weather is warm. The layer of air between the skin and the protective clothing soon becomes saturated with sweat, so that an artificial humid atmosphere is produced. If such clothing is essential for heavy work, its outside should be soaked in cold water. The evaporation of this water will cool down the worker inside.

In very hot conditions, as much as half to one pint of sweat may be lost per hour, and this must be made good by fluid intake.

Treatment

The patient should be

(a) removed from the heat;
(b) stripped to the waist and bathed or sprinkled with cold water;
(c) fanned with towels to encourage the evaporation of the water, which will cool the patient still further.

Medical or nursing help must then be obtained.

On recovery, the patient should rest quietly for a time, the length of the rest depending on the severity of the attack. All cases of heat exhaustion or heat stroke should be seen by a doctor or nurse before returning to work.

Sunstroke

This is usually a combination of heat exhaustion and ordinary fainting. It is particularly liable to occur in those who are suddenly exposed to the heat in unsuitable clothing. Its treatment is the same as for heat exhaustion (*see* above).

Rescue from burning buildings

If a fire is completely out of control, confine it to the burning area by shutting all doors to cut off the supply of oxygen.

The following rules should be observed in rescuing a patient from a burning building.

1 The rescuer should cover the nose and mouth with a cloth soaked in cold water. This helps to keep the hot overdried air out of the lungs.
2 The rescuer should crawl on hands and knees. Because hot air and smoke rise, the coolest and purest air is to be found nearest the floor.
3 The rescuer should feel any door before opening it. If it is very hot, it should be opened with great caution, so that he or she is not caught in a blast of hot air and flame.
4 The patient will probably be best moved by tying the hands together and hitching the arms over the rescuer's neck. The rescuer can then crawl along, pulling the patient's body below. Further details of the *neck-drag*, as this method of transport is called, will be given later (*see* page 157). If clothes catch fire, smother the flames with a coat or blanket.

Under normal circumstances only trained fire fighters are allowed to enter a burning room or building. First aiders should be aware of the company's fire drill and their own evacuation procedures.

Review questions

1   What is the immediate treatment of all minor burns?
2   When are burns serious? Why may they cause shock?

Also try the questions on burns on page 165.

8 Chemical injuries and poisons

Injuries and burns due to chemicals are far more common in industry than in domestic life. Chemical substances may harm the body in three ways:

(a) by directly burning the skin or eyes;
(b) by irritating the skin, so that dermatitis is produced;
(c) and by entering the body and causing rapid or slow poisoning.

Almost all chemical substances can cause trouble if misused. If used with understanding and proper care, however, they can be handled with complete safety. In this area in particular, prevention is better than cure, and in planning prevention management and workers must co-operate fully. This applies with equal force to measures for early and prompt treatment. Always make sure that workers follow manufacturer's instructions when using any chemical substances.

Chemical burns

Chemical burns may be caused by acids or alkalis. In either case, speedy treatment is vital. The acid or alkali must be washed off *at once*, or at least greatly diluted by flooding the affected part with large volumes of water. Thus, a chemical splash in the eye should be treated by holding the eye open under a running cold tap, or by plunging the upper part of the face into a bucket of cold water and blinking hard. Similarly, an acid or alkali splash on the skin should immediately be held under a running tap.

To lay people the word antidote has an almost magical significance. Hence there is always the danger that with chemical burns precious minutes may be lost hunting for an antidote, when speedy treatment with water will do far more good. The best antidote of all is plenty of water applied quickly. Only after this has been done should time be given to finding and applying the correct chemical antidote unless, of course, a large volume of antidote is immediately at hand.

In places where there are high risks, the provision of a shower cabinet is useful.

Acids

Acids may be quick-acting or slow-acting. The chief risks come from filling, transporting and emptying carboys, and from accidental spilling and splashing. Those without technical training for example, cleaners in laboratories, run special risks, and should be carefully instructed in the necessary precautions.

Quick-acting acids
With quick-acting acids the patient feels irritation and burning almost at once. Here are some examples of quick-acting acids.

1 *Hydrochloric acid* is used in pickling-vats, metal wire drawing, the manufacture of other acids, etc. It produces a dark brown blister which later turns black.
2 *Nitric acid* is a fuming liquid, acting even more quickly than hydrochloric acid. It is used in the chemical, explosives and pottery industries. It produces a yellow-brown skin burn.
3 *Nitro-hydrochloric acid* is a mixture, used for cleaning glassware.
4 *Sulphuric acid* is used in metal pickling, copper cleaning, and in the electric battery and chemical industries. It is similar in action to nitric acid.

Slow-acting acids
With slow-acting acids there is no immediate pain, so the patient may not know that he or she has been in contact with the acid for a period of half-an-hour to four hours. By then, the acid will have penetrated deep into the tissues. Here are some examples.

1 *Hydrofluoric acid*, a powerful and dangerous acid, is used for cleaning and etching glass, removing faults from pottery, and so on. The affected skin becomes dead-white. Inhalation of its fumes may produce ulcers inside the nose.
2 *Hydrobromic acid* is a similar but rather less powerful acid and is used in the photographic industry.
3 *Carbolic acid* and the phenols, cresols and lysols all act similarly.

Long contact may lead to burns or even absorption through the intact skin. The exposed skin is dead white and puckered.

4 *Oxalic acid*, used in printing, dyeing, leather and straw-hat making, is the slowest acting of the four. It affects particularly the fingers and may damage or destroy the nails. Similar damage around the nails may be produced by selenious acid, used in rectifier manufacture and for photo-electric cells.

Treatment of acid splashes

Again it must be emphasised that, with either type of acid, speed is vitally important.

1 Wash off the acid immediately with a large volume of water from a tap, shower or bath. Go on washing for at least ten minutes.

2 If tap water is not available, the acid should be washed off the skin with sterile water or saline which should always be available when chemicals are in use, and when there is no running water.

3 If the clothes are contaminated with acid, they should be removed at once if possible. If not immediately possible, the affected area of clothing should be flooded with water or a readily available antidote. If in doubt swill everywhere.

4 Slow-acting acids should be dealt with as above, but special treatment by a trained nurse or doctor will be needed to neutralise any acid which has penetrated into the tissues. For hydrofluoric acid splashes, after flooding with water and drying, *calcium gluconate gel* should be applied. This should be rubbed in gently to the area of the splash, and left on as a dressing while the patient is referred for medical treatment. Calcium gluconate gel, commonly called HF gel, should be kept in the first aid box wherever hydrofluoric acid is being used.

5 It follows that every suspected case of a slow-acting acid burn should be seen by a trained nurse or doctor as soon as possible after initial first aid treatment. With quick-acting acids, the same applies if, after initial treatment, the skin shows any change or the patient feels any adverse effects, or if the quantity of acid involved was at all considerable.

Prevention of acid burns

The prevention of burns is a matter for the management as a whole, often in consultation with the medical officer. This will include the provision of first aid facilities at all danger points. These will be described later when eye injuries are dealt with (*see* page 137). The medical officer must make sure that the workers and first aiders directly concerned know how to use these facilities.

Alkalis

Generally speaking, alkali burns are more serious than acid burns, because the alkalis tend to penetrate quickly into the tissues, and to go on acting even after thorough washing and neutralisation. Thus, alkalis closely resemble the more dangerous slow-acting acids. An alkali burn is therefore usually worse than it at first appears. Once the alkali has penetrated, the skin appears pallid and sodden, and later a deep slow-healing ulcer may develop.

The main alkalis used in industry are *caustic soda, caustic potash, ammonia, bleaching powder, lime* and *cement*. They are used in a wide variety of chemical processes, including the making of soap, paper, dyes and detergents, as well as for cleaning wool, barrels and enamel, and in the building industry.

Treatment of alkali splashes

First aid treatment is exactly the same as for acids, with the first emphasis on speedy complete washing with a large volume of water.

With lime, bleaching powder or cement, solid particles should be removed from the skin *before* the part is flooded with water, as water makes them stick. Removal is best done with a piece of cotton wool or a soft brush.

All alkali injuries should be seen by a trained nurse or doctor at the earliest possible moment. The provision of first aid facilities at danger points is even more important with alkalis than with acids.

Burns due to phosphorus, bromine and selenium

Rapid physical removal of any adhering solid particles should be followed immediately by thorough splashing with a large volume of tap water. The part should then be dried carefully, and the specific antidote in solution should be applied liberally on lint or gauze.

The specific antidotes are:

- for phosphorus, copper sulphate solution (3 per cent);
- for bromine, sodium thiosulphate solution (25 per cent);
- for selenium, sodium thiosulphate solution (10 per cent).

Tar burns

Burns caused by tar should be covered with a dry dressing and the patient referred to a trained nurse or doctor. Solidified tar is itself a good dressing, so no attempt need be made to remove it.

Chemical injuries to the eye

Eye injuries are dealt with initially in much the same way as chemical injuries to the skin, using large volumes of water, followed by an antidote as appropriate. They will be considered in detail later (*see* page 137).

Chemical skin irritation

Dermatitis or inflammation of the skin is a danger in industry. Almost any chemical substance can produce dermatitis in a person whose skin is sensitive, yet others can handle the same substances without danger. A strongly alkaline soap may also produce dermatitis. Some substances are particularly liable to cause trouble, for example:

- acids and alkalis;
- solvents and degreasers;
- detergents;
- oils and tars;
- glues;
- synthetic resins;
- plasticisers and accelerators;
- metallic irritants, such as mercury and arsenic;
- nickel and cyanide;
- sugar, flour and certain woods.

At the same time, it must be remembered that many skin complaints are not caused by occupation or chemical irritation of the skin. These non-industrial skin complaints are equally liable to lead to absence from work if neglected. They do not, of course, entitle the sufferer to industrial injury benefit.

Treatment

The first aider should never attempt to deal with a case of industrial dermatitis, or indeed any other skin condition, but can only encourage treatment by an expert at the earliest possible stage. Delay makes treatment far more difficult, and exposes others to the same risk.

Prevention

Prevention is a matter for the management and the doctor, and it must be individually planned wherever there is a real risk. It involves the proper planning of the job, the personal cleanliness of the worker and the use of a carefully selected barrier cream or other physical protection. Hence the proper hygiene of wash places and lavatories, and the changing and cleaning of protective clothing are of great importance. The first aider may have special duties here and may also help by directing the attention of the authorities to any possible hazard or risk. Remember that the most important single way of preventing industrial dermatitis is personal cleanliness.

Industrial dermatitis is not a *notifiable industrial disease* in the legal sense (*see* below) but the sufferer is entitled to claim under the Industrial Injuries Act (*see* page 183).

Chemical poisons

Chemical substances may enter the body through the skin, the lungs, or through the stomach and digestive system. The subject of industrial poisoning is a vast one, most of it being outside the range of the first aid worker. The first aider must, however, know how to deal with such emergencies as may arise and be aware of the existence of certain possibilities.

The direct action of chemicals on the skin has been dealt with above, but certain chemicals, for example chrome and nickel, may produce ulcers in the skin or in the membrane lining the nose. Such ulcers are known as *trade holes*. Fortunately these are now extremely rare. Certain other chemicals can penetrate the skin without damaging it. In consequence, they have to be handled with great care and, in these cases, safeguards are laid down by law.

Chemicals entering via the mouth, stomach and digestive system are of comparatively small importance in industry. More important, dirty hands may contaminate food. This emphasises the importance of washing the hands before food is eaten, and, where chemical processes are involved, of not eating in the vicinity.

Gases, fumes and dust

Gases, fumes and dusts are hazards in certain industries and are dealt with in detail later, as is asbestosis (*see* page 113). Many dusts, though unpleasant, are not poisonous. But dusts containing particles of silica of a certain size are liable, over the years, to produce severe lung damage. These risks are now well appreciated and the first aider should be aware of preventive measures.

Radioactive isotopes

Materials that are radioactive are widely used in industry, research, and in hospitals. Their use is closely controlled by regulations, and areas where they are stored or used have to be clearly marked with the international approved sign. Methods of handling should avoid contamination of the operator but an accidental spillage is always possible. Ingestion, inhalation, or skin absorption of radioactive chemicals will not only produce effects from the chemical itself, but also long term damage from the effects of radiation on the susceptible body tissues and organs. The severity of the effects will depend on the strength of the radioactivity – which varies from isotope (the technical name for a radioactive chemical) to isotope. Some are very weak, others are more hazardous.

Any contamination, whether of skin, clothes, wound or surroundings *must therefore be washed away as quickly as possible with large quantities of water* – which must also be collected and removed as it too will be radioactive. Detergent can be used on clothes, benches, and floor. All clothes, tissues, towels must be put into plastic bags and labelled for disposal. Washing must continue until the individual and surroundings can be monitored.

Advice must be obtained as soon as possible from the Radiation Safety Officer. Those responsible for helping with decontamination must wear full protective clothing.

Notifiable industrial diseases

As a result of the Factories Acts and the work of inspectors the well-known industrial poisons have been very largely brought under control. These poisons mainly cause symptoms of very slow onset, and are therefore seldom seen by the first aider at work.

Forty two different industrial diseases and conditions are notifiable by doctors and employers to the factory inspectorate of the Department of Employment (*see* page 182). If a first aider suspects either a process or an illness, he or she should let the occupational health department or the management know at once. The matter can then be investigated, and the Department of Employment medical advisor informed if there is a *prima facie* case for doing so. Chapter 16 *The legal framework* looks at notifiable diseases and claims for disablement benefit in more detail.

Review questions

1   How would you treat a man who spilt acid all over his overalls and bare arms?

2   How would you protect yourself against the risk of chemical splashes?

Also try the questions on chemical injuries on page 165.

9 Unconsciousness

The first aider who is faced with a patient who has been found, or has become, unconscious is not called on to make a diagnosis. He or she must, however:

- make an immediate assessment of what has happened; *and*
- at once decide if the patient is or is not breathing.

Most unconscious patients are still breathing. Check for breathing with the back of the hand or the cheek held near the patient's mouth and nose. If breathing has ceased, the patient is in immediate danger of asphyxia and urgently needs artificial respiration. Remember that unconsciousness and asphyxia (or suffocation) are different things, even though they may both be present at the same time. With unconsciousness, there may or may not be asphyxia. But with asphyxia, there is always unconsciousness. (*See* also chapter 10.)

Ascertaining the cause

There are three possibilities:

- (a) the cause is obvious;
- (b) it is probable;
- (c) the first aider can see no obvious cause.

It is vitally important to make an assessment, since the first step in first aid is to remove the unconscious person from danger, and this can be done only after a broad decision about the probable cause has been made.

Where the cause is obvious
Some circumstances in which the patient is found show fairly clearly what has happened – for example, where unconsciousness is due to partial drowning, electric shock, or head injuries.

In these circumstances the first aider must waste no time and save life if possible.

Where the cause is probable
In a situation where the cause of unconsciousness is probable we are concerned almost entirely with accidental gassing, whether domestic or industrial. Domestic gassing may occur in a bathroom, owing to a defective geyser, or in a bedroom, owing to a gas fire blowing out when the patient is asleep. Gassing in industry may have many different causes. *The first aider should know of risks in any particular processes in the workplace.*

Some common industrial processes always have a certain risk. Thus flues and boilers may develop defects, causing gas or exhaust to blow back into the work area; this may result in asphyxia or unconsciousness. Similarly, workers in deep holes and mines are subject to special risks.

No obvious outside cause
As a rule, the first aider will not be able to make an accurate diagnosis in cases where there is no obvious external cause. It will help to remember that there are six common causes, which cover most cases of this type:

- fainting;
- fits;
- strokes;
- diabetes;
- alcohol;
- hysteria.

These are discussed in detail on page 105.

Care of unconscious patients

Once the patient has been removed from external danger there are certain general lines of care, whatever the cause of the unconsciousness, which must always be followed.

1   Remove the unconscious person from danger. If he is *not* in danger do not attempt to move him.
2   Send for help, medical or nursing. If no nurse or doctor is immediately available, send for an ambulance. Give all essential information and accurate directions as to where the patient is.
3   Check the breathing:

(a) if possible look at the patient's chest, is it moving?
(b) listen close to the patient's mouth;
(c) feel the breath on your cheek.

If you suspect gassing, do not breathe in the patient's exhaled breath.

4 If the patient is breathing, roll him or her over into the recovery (*see* Fig. 5.2) or prone position (*see* Fig. 9.1). An unconscious patient may suffocate, if left lying on the back. The tongue falls back into the throat and may block the entry into the windpipe; so also may badly fitting false teeth. In addition, saliva or vomited material may be breathed into the lungs, with very serious results. Often the unconscious person is seen to be choking, struggling for breath, and turning blue. This may be due almost entirely to obstruction of the air passages, as a consequence of lying on the back.

Many lives have been lost because the patient has not been turned into the recovery or prone position. *Prone* means face downwards and the elbows bent, so that the forearms and hands are under the forehead (*see* Fig. 9.1). The *recovery* or *semi-prone* position means that the patient's body is on its side, face turned towards the ground. To stop the body rolling right over, the upper arm should be bent at the elbow and pulled up to support the shoulder. The upper leg must be bent at the knee, to support the hips. The lower arm is extended backwards behind the body and the lower leg is straight. Care must be taken to ensure that the lower shoulder is not pressed into the floor by the weight of the body (*see* Fig. 9.2). If there is retching or vomiting the recovery position is to be preferred as the mouth and nose are more easily kept clear.

Before rolling the patient over, make sure that no obvious fractures are present. If they are, roll the patient over but support the fractured part.

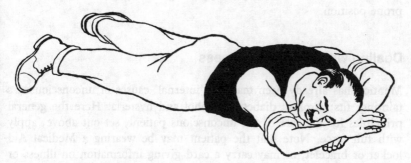

Figure 9.1 The prone position: note that the forehead and the chin are resting on the forearms and hands, and the face is turned very slightly to one side

Rolling should be done firmly but gently, moving the whole body into what looks like a natural and easy position.

5   Remove any false teeth. It is important to do this gently, so as not to injure the patient. If the jaw is tightly closed, do not try and force it open.

6   Raise the point of the chin with the hand, so that the neck is bent slightly back. This helps to open up the air passages at the back of the mouth. Try it on yourself, by dropping your chin on to your chest, and then lifting it well up; the difference in ease of breathing is immediately felt.

7   Loosen any tight clothing, especially round the neck or waist.

8   If the patient has to be moved, he or she should be lifted carefully on to a stretcher, still in the recovery or prone position, and carried in this way. Details will be given later (see page 149).

9   Make sure that all information and details of treatment are passed on to the medical or nursing staff, or to the ambulance crew.

Some don'ts

1   Do not force fluid (brandy, water or anything else) into an unconscious patient's mouth. The patient cannot swallow and will probably inhale it and may choke or get pneumonia.

2   Don't slap or throw water over the patient.

3   Don't try to transport the patient sitting up. He or she must be moved lying down in the recovery or prone position. Attempts to sit up an unconscious person, for example in the back of cars, can prove fatal.

4   If you suspect a fractured spine, because the patient has fallen from a height, or a weight has fallen directly on to the back, do not turn the patient over. If the patient is on the back, pull the chin well up and support it manually, keeping the airway clear. If he or she is on the front, turn the head sideways, supporting the chin on the arms in the prone position.

Dealing with unconsciousness

Mention has already been made of 'internal' causes of unconsciousness fainting; fits; strokes; diabetes; alcohol and hysteria. Here the general principles for the care of the unconscious patient, set out above, apply with full force. Note that the patient may be wearing a Medical Aid locket or bracelet, or may carry a card giving information on illness or treatment.

Fainting

Fainting has been discussed in detail on page 59. The unconsciousness is always of short duration.

Fits

Fits are alarming but are usually quickly over. They are almost always due to the condition of epilepsy, and the patient will often have had previous attacks. Happily, as a result of the new drugs used to control them, epileptic fits are much rarer than they used to be; but they may occur if the patient forgets to take the tablets or is overworked or under stress.

As a rule, at the start of the fit, the person utters a cry and then falls over. The limbs stiffen and then start to jerk. The patient may froth at the mouth, bite the tongue, pass urine or pass a motion. All the time the patient is quite unconscious, and when the violent phase is over falls into what appears to be a deep sleep. This usually lasts only a short time. The patient may be hurt in falling.

- Never restrain the patient violently. This simply makes the fit worse. The secret of good first aid is to prevent patients harming themselves. Pillows, coats, and other soft objects placed around the patient are safer and more effective than human strength.
- Never force the jaws apart in order to prevent tongue biting; it is possible to knock out teeth and fracture the jaw.
- Never tell an epileptic patient what the fit was like, as he may be quite unnecessarily distressed. Unconsciousness during the fit is one natural blessing of the disease.

After the attack is over, the patient should be advised to report to his or her own doctor as soon as possible.

Strokes

Strokes are caused by a bursting artery or a blood clot in the brain. Though a stroke is sometimes fatal, many patients recover. Good first aid care, as already described above, may save life.

The patient may feel giddy and may, or may not, pass out completely. As a result of the injury to the brain, the patient usually loses the ability to move one side of the body wholly or in part. This involves most obviously the arm or leg. At the same time, the other side of the face is also paralysed. In an unconscious patient who has had a stroke, the paralysed cheek may be seen flapping in and out each time the patient breathes.

The fact that the patient has had a stroke is suggested by:

1 the colour of the skin, which is usually blue;
2 age – patients are usually in their 50s or 60s;
3 loud, harsh breathing, called stertorous breathing;
4 the flapping cheek;
5 dribbling from the corner of the mouth.

Treatment is generally as set out above. Of course, the first aider must send for skilled help without delay.

Diabetes

Although people may wish to conceal the fact that they are diabetics, it is in their own interest that their condition should be known about, at any rate by the management or the medical department.

The most usual cause of trouble in a diabetic is overaction of a normal dose of insulin, as a result of physical fatigue, excessive work or worry, or missing a meal. The patient may become giddy, confused, and even apparently mentally disordered. The treatment is to give sugar at once, preferably in the form of a sweet drink. Skilled help should be sent for.

Alcohol

It must never be assumed that an unconscious patient who smells of alcohol is therefore drunk. People who feel giddy often take a drink before passing out. Tragedies can occur when an unconscious patient smelling of alcohol is handed over to the police. The proper course for the first aider is to send for expert nursing or medical help.

Hysteria

The first aider should never assume that an unconscious patient is hysterical. Indeed hysteria hardly ever causes complete unconsciousness.

Occasionally, however, a patient will become typically 'hysterical'. The situation is usually one of danger or anxiety, such as a manmade or natural disaster. Hysterical bad behaviour, like screaming or violent weeping, may lead to panic. In such circumstances, and in such circumstances only, firm physical measures are justified to prevent panic from breaking out.

More occasionally still, hysterical behaviour can follow serious injury to, or disease of, the brain. In these cases, it appears to be caused by lack of oxygen to the brain tissue. This is another reason why hysteria, other than the hysteria of panic, should be treated with gentle but firm kindness rather than the traditional slap.

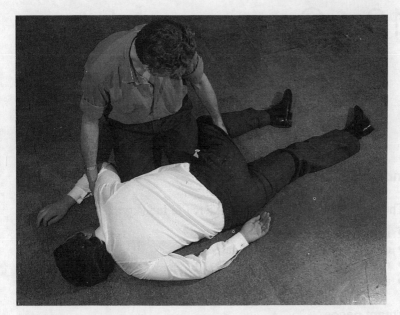

Figure 9.2   The recovery position. The patient has been rolled gently on to the side and the
first aider has bent the upper arm and leg to support the patient's shoulder and hips. The
lower arm is extended behind the body and the face is turned towards the ground so that
saliva and vomit can run out of the mouth and the airway can be kept clear

Review questions

1   What are some of the causes of unconsciousness?
2   What actions must you take if you are called to a person who has lost
consciousness?

Also try the questions on unconsciousness on page 165.

10 Gassing and asphyxia

Industrial gases

There are four types of gas encountered in industry:

- irritant gases;
- asphyxiating or smothering gases;
- tissue-poisoning gases,
- and narcotising gases

Irritant gases

Irritant gases are immediately detected by their effects, particularly on the nose and eyes. The smell is powerful, and the eyes start to water. The presence of the gas is so obvious that these gases are less dangerous than those which are non-irritant.

Table10.1 Irritant gases

Gas	Formula		Notes
Sulpher dioxide	SO_2	Manufacture of sulphuric acid; fumigation; refrigeration, etc	Also occurs in exhaust fumes and ordinary smoke
Ammonia	NH_3	Refrigeration, icemaking; other industrial processes	
Chlorine	CL_2	Bleaching; papermaking, etc	
Phosgene	$COCL_2$	Manufacture of some aniline dyes	Produced when trichlorethylene is inhaled through a lighted cigarette – hence those using trichlorethylene should not smoke at work

The common irritant gases met with in industry are shown in Table 10.1

Simple asphyxiating gases

The air we breathe consists of about four-fifths nitrogen and one-fifth oxygen. The nitrogen is inert; the oxygen is absorbed by the blood and carried throughout the body to enable the tissues to live; without oxygen the tissues die. Asphyxiating gases work simply by replacing the oxygen in the air. It follows that they must be present in very large quantities to get rid of enough oxygen to do harm. Most of them have no smell; this makes them the more dangerous. The common asphyxiating or smothering gases met with in industry are shown in Table 10.2.

Table 10.2 Simple asphyxiating gases

Gas	Formula		Notes
Nitrogen	N_2	Is important for practical purposes in wells, mines and other deep holes where all oxygen has been used up.	Absence of oxygen is shown when a safety lamp flame, lowered into the hole, goes out. In mines, nitrogen with some carbon dioxide (87% nitrogen + 13% CO_2) is spoken of as *black damp* or *choke damp*
Natural gas (North sea gas, petroleum gas) – a mixture of hydrocarbons, mainly methane	CH_4	In mines and domestic use, etc.	Known as *fire damp* as it explodes if ignited. Has no odour but for safety reasons an odour is added to domestic gas
Carbon dioxide	CO_2	Produced in living tissues as waste product and breathed out by lungs, produced in brewing, aerating and fermenting; common in mines	In mines, it is a constituent of *black damp*

Tissue-poisoning gases

Small quantities of tissue-poisoning gas exert a disproportionate poisonous effect. They are absorbed quickly into the blood from the lungs (or even the mouth) and equally quickly they poison the living tissues by preventing their intake of oxygen. The common gases under this heading are set out below.

Carbon monoxide (CO)

A constituent of coal gas, CO is also produced when coke, coal or petrol is burnt. In consequence, a blocked flue which causes the products of combustion to leak out into a workplace may produce carbon monoxide poisoning. The same result may be brought about by a petrol engine working in an enclosed space. Carbon monoxide may be met with in tunnels and at gas works and in coal mines, where it is called *after damp* because it follows explosions. Ordinary coal gas contains five per cent carbon monoxide; exhaust from a petrol engine seven per cent and producer gas 25 per cent.

Hydrogen sulphide or sulphuretted hydrogen (H_2S)

This gas evolved in glue making and tanning, and may occur in mines. In small concentrations it is violently irritating and has a foul smell, in large concentrations a man inhaling it may drop down dead. Because of its foul smell it is called *sink damp*. It may be produced accidently by the action of acids on sulphides.

Hydrogen cyanide (HCN)

HCN is so poisonous that it should never be employed except in the open air or in totally enclosed and extracted apparatus. Sometimes, however, it is used in the fumigation of premises or dirty fabrics. It has a smell of bitter almonds and is almost instantly fatal. Whenever it is used the official precautionary notice must be exhibited and the antidotes should be available. It may be produced accidently by the action of acids on cyanides.

Cyanide salts are equally poisonous if taken by mouth. Although they are widely used in industry for case hardening, and in solution for electroplating, casualties from their employment appear to be almost unknown.

Recent advances in the treatment of cyanide poisoning are outside the scope of first aid since they involve intravenous injections of an antidote called *kelcyanor*. This should be given by a doctor or specially trained nurse; side effects are liable to occur. First aiders can, however, administer *amyl nitrite capsules* which should be available wherever cyanides are used.

If an operator, while working with cyanide, collapses with giddiness or faintness, which may progress to loss of consciousness, the following action must be taken:

1 Remove the patient into the fresh air. Do not go into an enclosed space to rescue a patient without wearing appropriate breathing apparatus.
2 Check breathing and resuscitate if necessary. Do not breathe in the patient's exhaled air. If artificial respiration is required the *Holger Nielsen* method can be used (*see* page 123).
3 Crush an *amyl nitrite* capsule and hold it under the patient's nose for 15–30 seconds every two to three minutes. Make sure the airway is clear.
4 Call for a doctor or nurse, if available, immediately, and an ambulance at the same time. State that you suspect cyanide poisoning.

Narcotising gases

Narcotising gases produce anaesthesia or unconsciousness when inhaled, by acting directly on the brain. Many are used as anaesthetics in medicine. Any anaesthetic, if pushed too far, will ultimately prove fatal. Some industrial solvents have been used as anaesthetics, for example, ether and chloroform.

The most common anaesthetic used in industry is *trichloroethylene*, employed in degreasing. Workers in trichloroethylene tanks must be specifically instructed in the precautions needed to avoid gassing. A cautionary notice, usually provided by the makers, must be displayed and read.

There are many more degreasing and cleaning solvents used in industry and all of them are toxic if inhaled in excess. Safe handling rules should be taught and observed.

Symptoms of gassing

The symptoms of gassing depend on the nature of the gas, the amount inhaled and the length of exposure. With the irritant gases, coughing and watering of the eyes and nose are immediately apparent. With the tissue-poisoning and narcotising gases the patient quickly becomes unconscious but may retain a good colour. In the case of carbon monoxide and cyanide poisoning the patient may appear abnormally pink.

With the simple asphyxiating gases there are usually two stages.

(a) *Partial asphyxia*. The patient feels dizzy and weak and may stagger and collapse. There may be difficulty in breathing, with panting and gasping. Occasionally there are convulsions, especially as the patient breathes out.

(b) *Full asphyxia*. The patient is unconscious and blue, especially at the extremities – the nose, ears, lips and fingers. Breathing is at first intermittent and then absent. The pulse, too is first weak and then disappears. The absent pulse does not necessarily mean, however, that the heart has stopped.

Treatment of gassing

The treatment of gassing may be briefly summarised:

(a) removal from danger;
(b) artificial respiration if breathing has ceased (do not inhale the patient's exhaled breath, use the *Holger Nielsen* (*see* page 123) method if necessary);
(c) treatment of shock (*see* page 55);
(d) general care of the unconscious patient (*see* page 102).

Contaminated clothing should be removed as soon as possible. Medical advice and early treatment are essential, and if not available on site an ambulance must be called at once. The hospital must be informed of the name of the gas if this is known, and the full circumstances of the case. If the first aider has been trained in the use of oxygen, and it is available, it should be given.

Rescuing a gas casualty

As gas casualties are all too frequent in industry first aiders in where there are substantial hazards should be fully trained and practised in rescue work. The following are the general principles to be observed.

Never go into a gas filled area to rescue a patient without breathing apparatus, which should always be available where there is a risk of gassing. First aiders should know where the equipment is kept and how to use it.

1   Before entering a gas filled room or house, open, or if necessary smash, doors and windows, so as to get a through or cross draught. This will blow gas or fumes away. The first aider must be careful not to become a second casualty.

2 Remember that a damp cloth or towel tied round the face give *no* protection against gas.

3 If two or more people are present, one should stay outside in case the first needs help. A life line tied round the rescuer's waist should always be used. It is simply a rope, strong enough to pull a person along the ground.

4 If the rescue worker has to make a dash into a gas-laden atmosphere, he or she should take slowly six really deep breaths, then hold his breath and dash in. Most people can hold their breath for three-quarters of a minute to one minute at the most.

5 In gas filled places, the light is often poor. Some gases, for example carbon monoxide and methane, are inflammable. The first aider engaged in rescuing a gas casualty should *never* use a naked flame.

6 Respirators should not be used by the inexperienced or untrained first aider. Rescues which require their use also call for an experienced rescue worker. The proper use of respirators requires a good deal of practice. It is important to get specialist advice on the most suitable type of respirator for the work done, and to ensure that those wearing them are properly instructed and have plenty of practice. Details about the use of the different types of respirator are set out in the instructions issued by the makers of each type.

Dusts

Many industrial dusts are harmless, even if unpleasant. Some produce mild symptoms. A few are truly dangerous.

One of the slowly dangerous dusts is that from cotton fibre in textile mills. This produces a mild form of bronchial asthma called *byssinosis*. Exposure over many years may produce serious results.

Silica and asbestos

The most dangerous dusts are those containing silica, in the form silicon dioxide. This acts on the lungs to produce a hardening of the tissues which over the years is first disabling and may ultimately prove fatal. The condition is called *silicosis*. Common sources of silica are hard anthracite coals, flint chippings, and certain grinding processes. *Asbestos* is another dangerous source. It may give trouble during the manufacture of asbestos cloth, boarding, lagging and soundproofing materials, or if handling in any process or form which produces dust. Besides producing fibrosis or hardening of the lung, it can sometimes produce lung cancer.

Fumes

When melted, certain metals, such as cadmium and beryllium, give off dangerous fumes, and special precautions are needed. Fumes from other metals, such as copper, zinc and brass, if inhaled, can give rise to a sudden influenza-like illness called *metal-fume fever*. It can occur in both smelters and welders. Hence the need for good ventilation where these processes are carried out.

Isocyanates are increasingly used in the making of foam plastic and polyurethane. They can cause both bronchitis and bronchial asthma. Special extraction devices may be needed to safeguard exposed workers.

Dealing with dusts and fumes

Dust and fume suppression and control is a matter for the management, but the first aider can assist by example and precept in seeing that the workers concerned take the necessary precautions. This applies particularly to the use of filter-containing masks on dangerous processes.

Review questions

1   What kind of effects can gases have on those inhaling too much?
2   You are called to a laboratory when gas has escaped and a girl is inside and unconscious. What would you do?

11 Artificial respiration

When is artificial respiration needed?

Artificial respiration, or artificial breathing, is required *when breathing has stopped, but life is not extinct.*

Patients who need artificial respiration are always unconscious; but most unconscious patients have not stopped breathing, so do not need artificial respiration. The most usual causes of cessation of breathing are:

- electric shock
- drowning
- carbon monoxide poisoning
- pressure outside the chest, from falls of earth or masonry and, very rarely, from a dense crowd of people.

Why is artificial respiration needed?

In such cases, the time between the cessation of breathing and the stopping of the heartbeat is short. The purpose of artificial respiration is to give the heart and other tissues the oxygen they need, to remove the unwanted carbon dioxide from the body, and to encourage the lungs to start work again. Clearly, the speed is vital. Artificial respiration must be started on the spot, unless the patient has to be moved out of obvious danger, such as contaminated air.

Methods of artificial respiration

Many ways of carrying out artificial respiration have been devised. They may be considered under four main headings:

1 Push methods
2 Pull methods

3   Push and pull (Holger Nielsen) methods
4   Suck and blow methods

Push methods

In *push* methods the operator pushes on the outside of the chest to force
air out, relying on the natural recoil of the ribs to suck air in. The
classical push method is that of Schafer, which was invariably taught to
first aiders until a few years ago. It has the advantage of simplicity, but it
produces only a small movement of the lungs and cannot be used if the
ribs have been fractured.

Pull methods

In *pull* methods the operator moves the arms so as to stretch and expand
the chest thus causing an intake of air. The best known pull method is
that of Sylvester, although in this there is a small element of pushing as
well. Although Sylvester's method is now being taught as a useful
alternative to the mouth-to-mouth method, in our experience it is unsatisfactory. Since the patient is lying on his back, the airway is liable to
become blocked by the tongue, unless two trained first aiders are
present. Moreover, the arm movements are impossible for a small-build
first aider faced with a large patient. We therefore continue to teach the
Holger Nielsen method, below, as an alternative to the mouth-to-mouth
method.

Push-and-pull methods

Both the above methods are combined in push-and-pull methods. The
push-and-pull method devised by Holger Nielsen is now taught to first
aiders the world over. It is the most effective of the simple manual
methods, and will be described in detail later (*see* page 123).

Suck-and-blow methods

The lungs may be expanded and contracted in a natural way by applying
first a positive pressure, then a negative pressure, either outside the walls
of the chest or directly down the wind-pipe.

An outside pressure can be applied only with an elaborate mechanical
apparatus, the iron lung. It will never be available in first aid. It is,
however, of great value in hospital when the patient's breathing muscles
have been temporarily paralysed by a disease such as poliomyelitis.

Direct inflation and deflation of the lungs by air or oxygen is achieved by alternately blowing and sucking through the nose and mouth and the air passages. Provided there is a clear air way this method is completely effective. It is used by all modern anaesthetists during operations when chest and other muscles have been temporarily paralysed by special drugs. For first aiders, there are two possible suck-and-blow methods: mouth-to-mouth and use of a resuscitator

Mouth-to-mouth
The operator has to blow hard into the mouth of the patient, making sure that

1   the patient's chin is well up;
2   the mouth is open;
3   the tongue is out of the way;
4   the nostrils are closed; *and*
5   above all that there is a good fit of lips to lips.

The method is very effective and far easier to carry out than might be expected.

Using a resuscitator
Automatic resuscitators produce positive and negative pressure through a face mask, using no elaborate pumps or moving machinery. The power comes from the pressure of oxygen in an ordinary oxygen cylinder. Their full use is described in the manufacturer's booklet; properly employed, a resuscitator is the most efficient means of artificial respiration available to the first aider. We advocate their use in industry wherever there is a substantial risk of electric shock or asphyxia from other causes. Where a resuscitator is available, first aiders must receive special training in its use.

We are satisfied that for the great majority of patients the mouth-to-mouth method is now the first choice. If, however, the mouth or face are injured, the best method is the Holger Nielsen method. The first aider who is able to carry out these two methods efficiently, can do all that is generally required.

Practising mouth-to-mouth resuscitation

Every first aider should know how to perform mouth-to-mouth artificial respiration. It can be learnt from books or lectures; but the most valuable method is to practise on a special human dummy. The best teaching dummy available is: *Resusci-Anne*, available from:

Stores Manager
Laerdal Medical Ltd
see page 122, 172

This model is realistic and efficient. An attachment for teaching external heart massage can be obtained as an optional extra.

Even without the dummy, members of a family can practise on each other. There is much to be said for every boy and girl learning the method, so that if they are confronted with bathing accidents when no adults are present, they know what to do.

There are excellent films available, showing the practical details. An example is: *That they may live* (Canadian production from the University of Saskatchewan). It is available from:

Central Film Library
COI
Government Building
Bromyard Avenue
Acton
London W3

Carrying out mouth-to-mouth respiration

The details of the mouth-to-mouth method are as follows:

1   The patient lies on his *back* in the *supine* position. (Compare this with the Holger Nielsen Method where the patient lies on his face, in the prone position.)
2   Sweep a finger round inside the mouth, to remove weed, sweets, etc, and to make sure that the tongue is forward. Leave false teeth unless loose.
3   Kneel comfortably to one side of the patient's head, so that one's mouth can come naturally over the patient's.
4   Bend the patient's head right back, as far as it will go. This opens the air passage behind the tongue (*see* Fig. 11.1).
5   With one hand, hold the chin up and back. With the other, pinch the nose closed.
6   Take a deep breath. Apply your mouth to the patient's getting as good a fit as you can. Then blow, until out of the corner of your eye, you see the chest rise (*see* Fig. 11.2).
7   Remove your mouth, and watch the chest sink back.

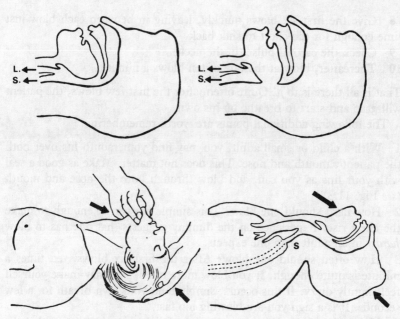

Figure 11.1   Mouth-to-mouth artificial respiration: position of head. (Top left) in the conscious person the back of the throat is clear so air can pass freely form the nose and mouth to the lungs (L is the windpipe leading to the lungs; S is the gullet leading to the stomach). (Top right) in the unconscious patieng lying on the back the tongue falls backwards, blocking the air passage. (Bottom) By bending the patient's head right back the air passage behind the tongue is once more opened

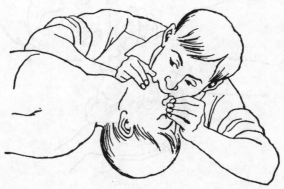

Figure 11.2   Mouth-to-mouth artificial respiration: positions for the first aider and patient. The first aider takes a deep breath and applies his or her mouth to the patient's and blows until the patient's chest visably rises. Throughout the patient's nose must be kept closed by pinching

8   Give the first six blows quickly, leaving in between each blow just time enough for the chest to sink back.

9   Check the carotid pulse (in the neck).

10   Thereafter, blow at the rate of ten blows a minute.

That is all there is to it. Quite often, after the first few blows, the patient will gasp and start to breathe on his own.

The following additional points are worth remembering:

1   With a child or small adult, you may find your mouth fits over both the patient's mouth and nose. This does not matter. Make as good a seal with your lips as you can, and blow through both the nose and mouth (*see* Fig. 11.3).

2   How hard should one blow? This simple answer is: enough to make the chest rise. Experience on the dummy suggests that one has to blow *harder* in an adult than one expects.

3   How often should one blow? After the first six blows, ten times a minute is quite enough. If you blow more often, you may make yourself feel slightly dizzy. If this occurs, simply hold your own breath for a few seconds. It is a sign you are blowing too fast.

4   If, in spite of your blowing, the chest fails to rise, it is a sign that the airway is blocked. This may be because:

(a) You have not got the chin back properly. Adjust, and try again.

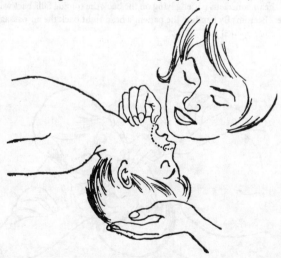

Figure 11.3   Mouth-to-mouth and mouth-to-nose artificial respiration. With a child or small adult the first aider's mouth fits over both the mouth and nose of the patient. Make as good a seal as possible with the lips and blow through both (the dotted line shows where the lips will fit)

(b) The patient's mouth will not open properly, because of muscle spasm, or will not stay open, because of flapping lips when the false teeth are out. You must then use the *mouth-to-nose* method. Apply your lips round the nose, making sure they do not block the nostrils. Keep the patient's mouth firmly closed, with your thumb on the lower lip, and still keep the chin well up and back. Then carry on as before. If the patient seems to have difficulty in breathing out, part his lips with your thumb each time.

(c) There is a blockage in the mouth. Have a look, and remove the blockage if you can.

(d) There is a blockage lower down in the throat or windpipe. If the patient is an adult, roll him or her into the semi-prone position, and give three sharp blows between the shoulders; again clear the mouth, roll the patient back to the supine position, and carry on. If the patient is a child, support him or her in the prone position across your knees with the head hanging down, or upside down by the heels, and give three sharp slaps between the shoulders. Again clear the mouth, and carry on.

5 Occasionally air enters the stomach as well as, or instead of, the lungs. If this happens, you can see the abdomen bulging out. Press gently over the stomach, when the air should come up with a gurgle. If food comes as well, clear it out with your finger before again starting mouth-to-mouth artificial respiration.

6 Carry on until natural breathing is going well. Time your blowing in to coincide with the patient's natural in-breathings. If the natural breathing is noisy or gurgling, clear the airway, and if this does not give relief, roll the patient into the semi-prone position.

The advantages of the mouth-to-mouth method are:

- it is less fatiguing than any other method of artificial respiration;
- it is the simplest and most effective method;
- it gives a much higher air intake into the patient's lungs than any other method
- it can be applied in awkward positions, for example when the drowned patient is still in the water, or when the body is trapped by a fall of earth.

The vital point to remember is to: **keep the chin well up, so as to give a good airway**.

Questions and answers

Here are some of the questions first aiders usually ask.

Is expired air from one's lungs as good as natural air?
Natural air contains about 20 per cent oxygen. Expired air contains about 16 per cent of oxygen. This is quite enough to saturate the patient's blood with oxygen.

What about water in the patient's lungs?
This appears to matter much less than we once thought. In drowning, comparatively little water actually gets down into the lungs, because of spasm in the voice-box or glottis. Provided the heart is functioning, the water is very quickly absorbed from the lungs by the blood. The water which sometimes gushes from a drowned person's mouth is mainly from the stomach.

Is there any danger of infection in the method?
The risk is very slight unless there is contamination by blood *and* the patient is infected *and* the first aider has a wound on the lip. Plastic protectors can be purchased which give complete protection when placed over the patient's mouth.

1   *Resusci Ade*: this has to be used very carefully as the mouthpiece is rather small. The use of this aid must be practised and care must be taken to make an airtight seal around the nose and mouth when blowing in through the mouthpiece, but relaxing the seal during the expiration phase so that the patient's exhaled air can escape between the mouth and the plastic sheet. It is available from:
Portex Ltd
Hythe
Kent.
2   *Laerdal Pocket-mask*: this is a plastic face piece which covers the patient's nose and mouth with a mouthpiece through which the first aider blows. Exhaled air passes out through a one-way valve at the side. It is easy to use and can be obtained from Laerdal Medical Ltd (*see* page 27).
3   *Bioglan Microshield (disposable)*: this resembles *Resusci Ade* but has a larger mouthpiece. It is available from Bioglan Laboratories Ltd (*see* page 27).

All masks must be disinfected after use as described in Chapter 2 (*see* page 26).

Will the method work in gas poisoning cases and is there then any risk to the first aider?
It will work, and there is no risk. Remember again that the first aider is blowing out. The amount of poison gas the patient will breathe out is

negligible. Of course, the patient must be removed into a gas-free atmosphere before artificial respiration is started.

What about aesthetic objections?
These do not arise in practice. If you like, you can put a handkerchief over the patient's face, and breath through this. This method works quite satisfactorily. But it is unnecessary.

Carrying out the push-and-pull or Holger Nielsen method

Preparation

Before starting the push-and-pull, or Holger Nielsen method, the following steps should be taken as quickly as possible.

1 Roll the patient into the prone position.
2 Put the finger inside the mouth and sweep it around to remove any obstruction – for example, sea or pond weed or loose false teeth.
3 Make sure that the tongue is hanging in its normal forward position.
4 Loosen the collar.
5 Remove any 'lumps' in the clothing from the front of the chest – for example, a tin in a pocket. Such an object may damage the ribs when artificial respiration is started.
6 If the patient has been submerged or has been vomiting, the first aider should stand astride the patient, clasp the hands underneath the patient's stomach and raise the patient quickly a short distance from the ground. Repeat twice. This helps to empty the air passages.
7 Do not waste any time in removing wet clothing.

These steps should not take more than a minute or so. Artificial respiration should then be started immediately. Meanwhile an assistant should send for a doctor and an ambulance and make arrangements for an automatic resuscitator if this is available.

Artificial respiration should be continued rhythmically without stopping, until natural breathing starts again, or until the doctor pronounces the patient to be dead. Remember that patients have sometimes been revived after as long as an hour or more. When the patient begins to breathe without help, the timing must be adjusted to fit in with the breathing. From then on, the patient sets the rhythm, and the first aider has to help the patient's own chest movements. Once the patient is breathing properly, he or she should be well covered and left lying quietly in the prone position until removed by ambulance to hospital.

Technique in the Holger Nielsen method

The Holger Nielsen method is also known as the *back-pressure arm lift* method, a good descriptive title as we shall see.

Position
The patient must be placed in the *prone* position (*see* Fig. 9.1) with the elbows bent and projecting out sideways and the hands crossed under the head. The head will be turned slightly on one side so that the cheek rests on the hands. The nose and mouth must be clear of any obstruction.

1   Kneel on one knee at the head of the patient and facing him or her. Place the knee in the angle between the patient's head and forearm. Place the opposite foot near the patient's other elbow. (*See* Fig. 11.4). Alternatively, kneel on both knees, one on either side of the head. If the one-knee position is used, it is best to change the knee from time to time.

2   Places your hands on the flat of the patient's back. The tips of the thumbs should be just touching, with the fingers pointing downwards and outwards and the wrists on a level with the armpits (*see* Fig. 11.5).

3   In making the movements, your arms should be kept straight and the body weight used to produce the effects. All the movements should be made steadily, slowly and rhythmically, counting out loud slowly as you proceed.

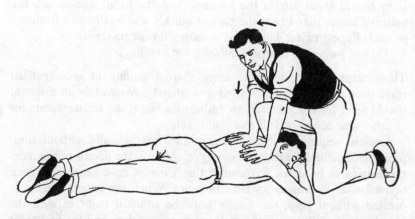

Figure 11.4   Holger Nielsen method of artificial respiration: the position of the first aider and patient at the start of the cycle. Note the patient's head is turned slightly to one side with the cheek resting on the hands. The first aider's knee is in the angle between the patient's head and the forearm; the first aider's arms are straight, inclined at an angle to the patient's back

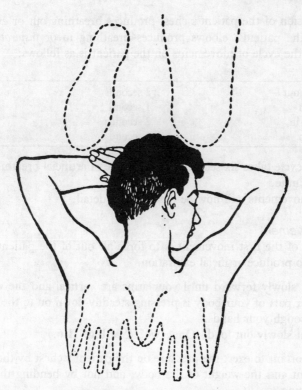

Figure 11.5 Holger Nielson method: position of the first aider's hands on the patient's back. Note that the tips of the thumbs are just touching and the wrists on a level with the patient's armpits

Movements

The sequence of movements is best looked at first in tabular form as in Table 11.1.

Table 11.1 Sequence of movements in the Holger Nielsen push-and-pull method

Movement	Time	Count
First movement:		
Compression of patient's chest	2 seconds	'One, two'
Second movement:		
Slide hands to patient's elbows	1 second	'Three'
Third movement:		
Raise patient's elbows	2 seconds	'Four, five'
Fourth movement:		
Lower elbows and slide hands to patient's back	1 second	'Six'

Compression of the patient's chest produces breathing out or *expiration*. Raising the patient's elbows produces breathing in or *inspiration*. The effect of the cycle of movements on the patient is as follows:

Breathing out	2 seconds
Relaxation	1 second
Breathing in	2 seconds
Relaxation	1 second

The full cycle takes six seconds, giving a rate of artificial breathing of ten to the minute.

The movements will now be described in detail.

First movement

The aim of the first movement is to force air out of the patient's chest, that is, to produce artificial expiration.

1 Rock slowly forward until your arms are vertical and the weight of the upper part of your body is pressing steadily down on to the patient's chest through your hands.

2 Count slowly out loud: 'One, two'. (*See* Fig. 11.6.)

It is important to exert the pressure on the patient's chest by the rocking movement and the weight of the body, and not by bending the elbows and pushing.

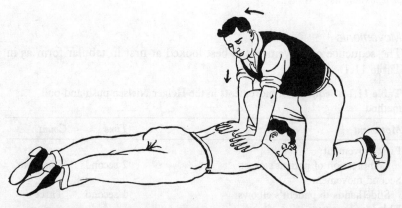

Figure 11.6 Holger Nielsen method: first movement in cycle – compression of the chest producing artificial expiration (breathing out). The first aider has rocked forward, so the arms are vertical and the elbows are kept straight. The weight of the first aider's body is pressing steadily down on the chest

Second movement

3 Relax the pressure on the chest wall and rock slowly backwards, sliding your hands up the patient's arms to just below his or her elbows.
4 Count out loud: 'Three'. (*See* Fig. 11.7.)

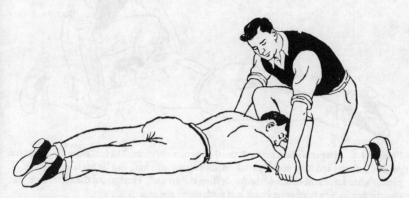

Figure 11.7 Holger Nielsen method: second movement in cycle. The first aider has rocked backwards, sliding the hands and arms (still straight) along the patient's arms to the elbows. The release of pressure on the chest has already started the process of inspiration (breathing in)

Third movement

The aim of the third movement is to stretch the chest so as to draw in air, thus producing artificial inspiration.

5 Draw the patient's elbows and arms up off the floor, towards you.
6 Count out loud 'four, five'. (*See* Fig. 11.8.)

In making this movement it is important not to drag the patient's body forward towards the operator; this tends to bend up the neck and block the airway.

Fourth movement

7 Drop the patient's arms gently to the ground.
8 Slide your hands down the arms and back to their starting position on the chest. Counts out loud: 'Six'. (*See* Fig. 11.6.)

General points

How hard should the operator press on the chest? This must vary with the build and size of the subject. For a large male, pressures of 30 lb may be exerted; for a small female 12 lb and proportionately less for a child.

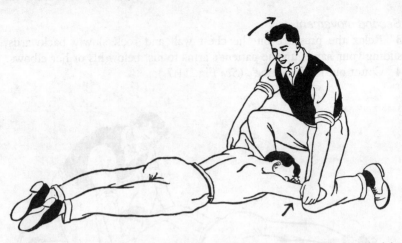

Figure 11.8   Holger Nielsen method: third movement in cycle. The first aider has raised the patient's elbows and arms and drawn them slightly towards him. But he has not raised the patient's head from the hands or the hands from the ground. Throughout the cycle, note the way the first aider's head moves back and forth above the patient

To estimate these pressures, try pressing on a bathroom spring-weighing machine. A strong man must be careful not to do damage by pressing too hard on a small subject.

When breathing starts, the arm-raising and lowering only should be carried out, keeping carefully in time with the breathing. Count 'one', 'two', 'three', for inspiration when the arms are raised, and 'four', 'five', 'six' for expiration when the arms are lowered.

If there are chest injuries, the first movement of pressing on the chest should be omitted and arm-raising and lowering only should be carried out. If there are arm injuries, the arms should be laid by the sides. The chest-pressure movement should be carried out, but in place of the arm and elbow-raising, the points of the shoulders should be lifted from underneath. If there are chest injuries and arm injuries, shoulder-raising only should be carried out.

Oxygen

Although oxygen is not necessary for first aiders' use, it may be available when its use is supervised by a doctor or nurse.

Oxygen resuscitation apparatus consists:

- of a cylinder containing compressed oxygen;

- a main valve (often spanner-operated);
- a control valve;
- a pressure-gauge;
- a corrugated rubber or stiff plastic tube; *and*
- a face mask.

Certain models embody a flow meter and a flexible rubber breathing bag. In some, the flow of oxygen to the mask is governed by the movements of the breathing bag, and hence by the movements of the lungs. In others, the flow to the face mask is regulated by the control valve.

As the details for operating each type of machine vary, first aiders must study and master the manufacturer's instructions before use.

In applying any type of face mask to a patient, it is important that the chin should be raised up from the neck as much as possible, so as to maintain a good air way. The mask can be applied and the chin raised with one hand, with the little finger under the chin. The details of the method are best learnt by demonstration and practice.

Cardiopulmonary resuscitation (CPR)

If the heart has ceased to move the blood around the body artificial respiration is no use. It is sometimes possible to restart the heart by pressing over the lower half of the sternum or breast-bone. This is *external heart or cardiac massage*, and if after six breaths with the mouth-to-mouth method the patient still looks dead – that is, there is no change in the colour of the skin or lips and no signs of spontaneous breathing movement, feel for the carotid pulse. If you cannot feel any pulse and you are confident you know how to feel it, you may try cardiac massage.

Technique

(a) Place the ball of one hand over the lower half of the breast bone. This will be found at the top of the inverted V made by the lower ribs.

(b) Place the second hand over the first.

(c) Give six sharp presses at one second intervals (*see* Fig. 11.9).

(d) Give two mouth-to-mouth lung inflations.

(e) Repeat the whole cycle but give 15 presses followed again by two inflations.

(f) Stop the external heart massage as soon as the colour improves, but continue with the mouth-to-mouth artificial respiration.

If two first aiders are available one can give heart massage while the other

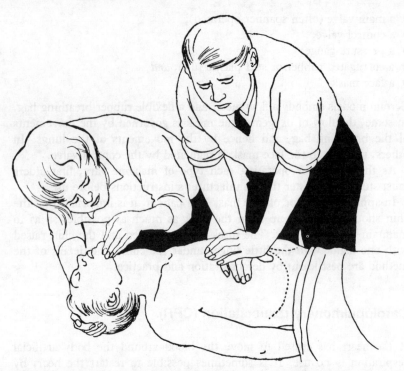

Figure 11.9   Mouth-to-mouth method with cardiopulmonary massage. If after six mouth-to-mouth breaths the patient still looks dead, external heart massage should be tried. Six sharp presses are applied over the lower half of the breast bone, at one-second intervals. A mouth-to-mouth breath is then given, and the cycle of presses and breathing is then repeated

gives mouth-to-mouth artificial respiration. One ventilation to five compresses.

With a child or infant, two fingers over the lower half of the sternum will give sufficient pressure.

Review questions

1   Describe how you would carry out mouth-to-mouth respiration.
2   When would you not use mouth-to-mouth? Describe another method of artificial respiration.

12　The eye

Frequency of accidents

Far too many accidents in industry involve the eye; by far the commonest of these is a foreign body in the eye. It is obvious that eye injury constitutes a most important part of the first aider's work.

Most industrial eye casualties never reach hospital but are dealt with by first aiders, industrial nurses, industrial medical officers, or general practitioners. Nevertheless, one third of all patients going to an eye hospital come from industry. Most industrial eye casualties come from turning, milling, spinning, boring, hammering and chipping.

Examining the eye

Any first aider who may be called upon to deal with a colleague's eye should know how to examine it. This is best taught in a first aid class by each examining the eye of a fellow student.

1　The patient should be seated, with a good light shining on the face and eye. The first aider should stand behind the patient and support the head against his or her own body.
2　The patient's head should be tipped well back and the eye then held open with two fingers (see Fig. 12.1). It will make it much easier to examine the bad eye if the patient is asked to keep both eyes open. The patient should be made to look slowly and in turn at each of the four points of the compass, so that the whole of the exposed eye may be carefully inspected. There should be no hurry. It is particularly important to inspect the front of the cornea (the transparent curved surface covering the pupil and iris).
3　If nothing can be seen, the lower lid should be pulled away from the globe while, at the same time, the patient looks upwards. This enables the first aider to spot any foreign bodies under the lower lid. It is

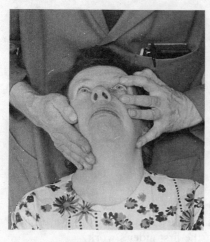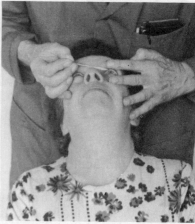

Figure 12.1 Examining an eye. The first aider stands behind the patient supporting the head against his or her own body. The patient's head is tipped well back and the eye held open with two fingers of the left hand

Figure 12.2 Removal of a foreign body with a cotton wool applicator: note that the eye is held open with the left hand while the applicator is held in the right hand

possible to turn up the upper lid in such a way that its under surface can be seen, but as this manoeuvre needs considerable experience if it is to be satisfactorily performed, it is best not done by first aiders.

A foreign body may be seen:

- on the front of the cornea;
- on the white of the eye;
- on the red inside lid.

It may be black or glistening, and may be fixed or moving.

Removal of a foreign body

A foreign body which moves will probably come out of the eye very easily. Nature's method is to flush the eye with tears from the tear-gland. Flushing can be produced by getting the patient to blow his nose strongly, and blinking several times. On no account must the eye be rubbed.

Using water

Should this fail the eye should be washed out with running water–tap water, sterile water or saline. (*See* page 137 for treatment.) If this fails to remove the foreign body, then it is almost certainly stuck to the surface of the cornea.

Using cotton wool

The first aider who feels confident and has been properly instructed may make one attempt, and one only, to remove a foreign body which fails to come away with washing. But if expert medical or nursing help is readily available, it is better to pass the patient on for skilled attention.

The attempt at removal should be made with clean cotton wool on an applicator (*see* Fig. 12.2). In the Harlow first aid box, six of these are provided (*see* page 19). When one has been used it should be thrown away immediately. The eye should be held open and a single sweep with the cotton wool should be made over the foreign body. If it is loose, it will be seen attached to the tip of the cotton wool. To make sure that the foreign body has gone, the eye should be carefully inspected under a good light.

The first aider should *never* use the corner of a handkerchief. It will not be sufficiently clean to be safe. A camelhair brush is also unsatisfactory because it is too soft; moreover, if not sterilised after use, it will carry germs from eye to eye.

Referral

Unless the first aider is completely certain that a foreign body has been removed, the patient should be referred to a nurse or doctor at once. If the patient complains of any pain at all after removal, this also is an indication for referral.

A foreign body so well embedded in the surface of the cornea that it does not project may at first cause no pain. There may be a latent period before the onset of pain of up to twelve hours, or occasionally even longer. Any patient who complains of pain and thinks that the foreign body entered at some earlier time should therefore be referred straight away to a nurse or doctor.

If a foreign body has been in the eye for some time, it may leave behind a small red ring of rust. A nurse or doctor will remove this quite easily the following day, after the foreign body has been dealt with. It cannot be removed by a first aider.

It is essential that the first aider should run no risks in dealing with eye injuries. If there is the slightest doubt, the patient should be sent to a nurse or doctor at once. This applies with special force at night, when there may be natural reluctance to call a doctor on duty. Always cover the eye with a medium-sized dressing or eye-pad before referral.

A doctor or sister can make use of a local anaesthetic on the eye, so that both examination and treatment can be slowly and thoroughly carried out. No eye drops or ointment should ever be inserted by a first aider.

Glass in the eye

It may be very difficult to see glass in the eye. Moreover, a piece of glass is liable to cut the surface of the eye, sometimes severely. The first aider must not wash out the eye, for fear of the washing fluid getting into the globe through the cut. The first aider should not attempt to remove glass from the eye. The eye should be covered with a medium-sized individual sterilised dressing, and the patient sent for expert treatment as quickly as possible. Only if there has been a chemical splash into the eye as well as glass must the first aider very gently wash out the eye before covering and referral.

Dust in the eye

Dust may blow into the eye in workshop areas or be blown up following the use of a compressed air hose for clearing debris. The eye should be washed out, using water (*see* page 137). If the irritation is not speedily relieved, the patient should be sent to a nurse or doctor, in case there is a scratch on the cornea.

Scratches of front of eye

The cornea or the conjunctiva (the membrane covering the white of the eye and the inside of the eye-lids) may be scratched by a brush of the hand or some other object. The patient often thinks there is a foreign body in the eye, but on examination the first aider will usually be unable to see anything abnormal, though there may be a good deal of watering. Such cases should always be referred to the nurse or doctor for treatment as these scratches may otherwise become infected, leading to the painful and much more dangerous condition of corneal ulcer.

Foreign bodies within globe of eye

A foreign body which penetrates the globe of the eye will not be visible when the eye is examined, though a small cut in the cornea or the white of the eye may be seen. Such an accident usually follows hammering or chiselling with a badly worn chisel. A part of the head flies off at high speed and penetrates completely. Any eye accident following the use of a chisel or hammer must be assumed to be serious, and should be sent for immediate treatment. The eye should be covered with a medium-sized individual sterilised dressing and the patient should be transported by car or ambulance; movement of the head and upper part of the body must be kept to a minimum for fear of starting bleeding within the eyeball. In such a case, it is dangerous to wash out the eye.

If it is not swiftly diagnosed and treated, the patient may lose the use of an eye.

Conjunctivitis

Conjunctivitis is the state of inflammation of the membrane covering the front of the eye and the inner sides of the eyelids. The patient feels a pricking or irritation in the eye and the eye itself appears red. The condition may be caused by germs or dust, but in industry there is often a foreign body present, the entry of which has not been noticed by the patient. For this reason it is best to refer every case of conjunctivitis to a trained nurse or doctor for investigation. In industry, conjunctivitis may also be caused by chemical fumes.

Haemorrhage under conjunctiva

It is appropriate here to mention the haemorrhages which sometimes occur under the conjunctiva. The whole of one side of the white of the eye is red, giving a somewhat alarming appearance, but the patient feels nothing abnormal. Usually a sub-conjunctival haemorrhage is not at all serious, but nevertheless it is a wise precaution to refer all such cases to a doctor.

Welding and the eye

Exposure of the unprotected eye to gas or electric welding or cutting is the commonest cause of conjunctivitis in industry. There are three common types of welding:

- spot welding
- gas welding
- electric arc welding

Spot welding

The operator ought to wear goggles or have the eyes protected with a mica or other transparent shield. The only risk to the eye is from sparks. Eye injuries from spot welding should be referred for expert treatment, as tiny pieces of metal are usually stuck to the burnt conjunctiva.

Gas welding

Oxygen (4,000 degrees Fahrenheit) and acetylene (6,000 degrees Fahrenheit) are the common flames used.

Electric arc welding

The temperatures here are similar to those with gas welding. The welding rod is one electrode, and this melts to fill the space between the metals to be welded.

Both gas welding and electric arc welding produce ultra violet light. This is harmful to the eyes and will cause acute inflammation of the conjunctiva. Welding or cutting places should be well ventilated, as certain harmful gases are present; they should also be screened to prevent exposure to these strong ultra-violet rays.

Arc-eye or welder's flash

Welder's flash follows exposure of the unprotected eye to gas or electric welding or cutting. The operator must use dark goggles or a dark shield and most operators are fully aware of this. The main risk is to others in the vicinity, such as fellow workers and trainees. Momentary exposure is enough, and trouble can be caused up to 200 feet away, especially if exposure is prolonged.

The condition resembles snow blindness: the eye is red, watery and uncomfortable, and the patient will usually remember momentary exposure to a welding flash four to eight hours previously. When there is no such recollection, it may be impossible for the first aider to distinguish this condition from a foreign body.

For safety, all cases of arc-eye should be referred for treatment. The first aid treatment is to wash out the eye with water or a simple solution, but a special *arc-eye lotion* and other special preparations are more effective. These preparations however, are best applied by a trained nurse. Dark glasses give some relief.

Exposure of the unprotected eye to infra-red rays from furnaces, molten glass or white-hot metal can, over many years, damage both the lens and the cornea. The result is opacity of the lens or cataract. Modern methods of protection have virtually eliminated this condition.

Chemical splashes in the eye

In dealing with chemical splashes, first aid is of the utmost importance, since it can, if done promptly and efficiently, save sight. As with chemical burns of the skin, alkalis are more dangerous even than acids (*see* page 96). Unless the alkali is removed at once, it combines with the tissues of the eye and goes on acting on the tissues long after the eye has been thoroughly washed out. A neglected alkali burn of the eye will in consequence continue to increase in size and depth despite washing with antidote, and this may cause loss of vision.

The common alkalis liable to get splashed into the eye are: caustic soda, ammonia (especially from refrigerator plants), lime and cement. Other liquids used in industry which may get into the eye are the industrial acids, mentioned earlier, thinners, solvents and de-greasers. Although these should all be flushed out as quickly as possible, they are less likely than alkalis to cause permanent damage.

Treatment

(a) Hold the head under a tap, over an eye irrigation tap (a drinking fountain works quite well), or under a container of sterile water or saline.

(b) make the patient blink vigorously.

The patient may have difficulty in opening the eye because of spasm and should be told to try to hold both eyes open. If the first aider is trying to irrigate the eye with water sterile water or saline, the patient should sit or lie with the head tilted right back and an assistant should hold the eye open; if no assistant is available, the first aider may use the first and second fingers of the left hand. The jet of water or saline should not be directed right on to the front of the eye; instead, the patient should be told to look outwards and the jet directed on to the inner angle of the eye (*see* Fig. 12.3). Every occupational first aider should have experience of irrigating an eye, both giving and receiving; there are few more useful class exercises.

Wherever there is a high risk of chemical splashes, sterile eye wash should be readily available in containers with an irrigating nozzle that usually needs to be cut to release the flow of water (*see* Fig. 12.4).

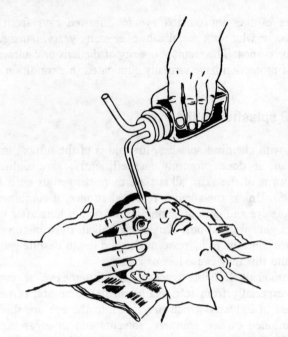

Figure 12.3 Washing out the eye following a chemical splash. The irrigating bottle is held in the left hand and the eye is held open

Irrigation should be continued, with short rest pauses for the patient, for five to ten minutes. The patient should then be transferred, as swiftly as possible, to expert nursing or medical care, for inspection and further irrigation if necessary. After alkali splashes, this irrigation may have to continue for longer.

Contact lenses

It is important that anyone handling chemicals should wear protective glasses, but it is doubly important that those who wear contact lenses should do so. If a chemical gets into the eye the lids may go into spasm and it may be difficult to get the lens out. The chemical will be trapped under the lens and will be more liable to injure the eye.

If the lens has not come out with the first washout then the first aider must persuade the patient to put the eye right under water in any clean bowl or basin that is available and open the eye under water, moving the eyeball round at the same time. Because of the spasm the first aider will have to exercise considerable persuasion and help the patient to open the

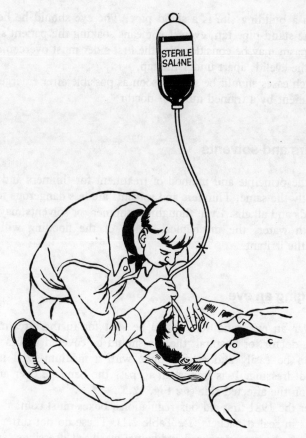

Figure 12.4 Washing out the eye using sterile saline from a container suspended from a wall hook. These containers have a tube and nozzle which can easily be cut or broken when a jet of saline (or sterile water) gushes out. The patient is lying flat on the floor with the head on a piece of newspaper; the eye is held open and the jet of saline is directed into the inner angle of the eye

eye. Do not be deterred by fears of losing the lens, most are insured, but if not, the eye is more precious than the lens.

Lime or cement in the eye

The principle of treatment for lime or cement is just the same as for other splashes. Flood the eye with water or salt solution immediately and go on flooding for at least five minutes. Speed is vital. Often the only source of water on a building site is a stand pipe. The eye should be held open under the stand-pipe tap, even if it means soaking the patient's clothes. Eyelid spasm may be considerable; the first aider must overcome this by pulling the eyelids apart under the tap.

All such cases should be seen as soon as possible after emergency first aid treatment by a trained nurse or doctor.

Thinners and solvents

Again, the principle and method of treatment for thinners and solvents are exactly the same. Thinners and solvents are less dangerous to the eye than acids and alkalis. Even though the thinners or solvents may not mix well with water, the mechanical action of the flooding will quickly remove the irritant.

Bandaging an eye

Whenever an eye condition has to be sent for further treatment to a nurse, a doctor, or hospital, the eye should be covered with a bandage. This can be easily and swiftly done with a medium-sized individual sterilised dressing. It is important to pass the bandage over and under the ear on the affected side (see Fig. 12.5).

Under the 1981 first aid box regulations, boxes must contain sterilised eye-pads in sealed packets (see Table 2.1). These do not differ substantially from the medium-sized individual sterilised dressings, and either may be used to cover an eye in exactly the same way.

Prevention of eye injuries

If safety spectacles or protective face-shields were more widely worn in industry, eye injuries, whether from chemical splashes or foreign bodies, would be far fewer. There may be a traditional reluctance in certain factories to wear safety spectacles, or, where the need is only occasional, they may be forgotten. Sometimes, unsuitable goggles mist up and prevent the proper performance of the job; a face-shield, which is not closely applied round the eyes, may be the answer. It is unrealistic to expect workers to wear goggles when the risk to the eyes is slight. But when the risk is great, not to protect the eyes is extremely dangerous.

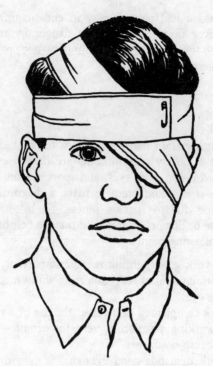

Figure 12.5   Medium-sized individual sterilised dressing used as an eye-bandage. Note that the bandage passes above and below the ear on the injured side. The method of applying the official sterilised eyepad is precisely the same

Here are some practical points about the relative dangers of different processes and materials

- Grinding wheels should always be eye-guarded, either by transparent plastic shields fitted to the mountings, or by the wearing of goggles.
- Some metals fracture more easily than others and therefore shoot off dangerous particles when worked; examples are aluminium and magnesium alloys, and bronze. Mild steel flies more than cast iron.
- A continuous cutting lathe is less dangerous than one with an intermittent cut, because continuous swarf does not usually fly.
- Fettling and milling with an interrupted cutter are both potentially dangerous.
- Flying particles of wire can be very dangerous, but when trimmed, some types of wire fly more than others. Another wire danger arises when particles fly off wire brushes used for cleaning structural steel.

The first aider has a real part to play in encouraging the use of eye protectors whenever there is substantial danger by making sure that workers appreciate the risks they are running by not protecting their eyes on the more dangerous jobs.

Eyestrain

Complaints about eyestrain may be made to the first aider. The patient may believe that a variety of symptoms are due to eyestrain, such as headaches, blurred vision, sore eyes, and spots in front of the eyes.

The first aider is not competent to make a diagnosis – many of the symptoms may be due to specific illness. Such complaints must be referred to a nurse or doctor. However, it may be helpful if the first aider is aware of the following points:

- whatever the work good lighting is most important, without glare or flicker, and without a lot of reflection from shiny surfaces, all of which can irritate the eyes.
- where the work complained of involves the use of a visual display unit (VDU), the working position is very important – neck strain, for example, can cause headaches.
- where the work demands good eyesight, (e.g. with a microscope, a magnifying glass, or a VDU) the operator needs to have his or her eyesight properly tested and corrected if necessary by glasses. Properly organized work will not cause eyestrain if the vision is good enough for the work to be done.

Review questions

1 How do you examine an eye?
2 A girl with a contact lens gets an acid splash in her eye, what do you do?

Also try the questions on the eye on page 166.

13   Common ailments

Distinguishing major and minor ailments

In dealing with illness as opposed to injury, the first aider is in much the same position as the parent in the home. The first aider must resist the temptation to try to become a semi-skilled doctor – the job is to make not diagnoses but rather some simple practical decisions:

- Is the condition a minor one, which will get better quickly at work?
- Is the patient sufficiently ill to be sent to the surgery or industrial health centre, or, if these are not available, to be sent home?
- Is the patient so ill that skilled help must be sent for at once?

The major emergencies at work have already been dealt with, and the first aider should be able to recognise shock (even when caused by internal trouble such as stomach bleeding or a heart attack and not by an accident), strokes and epilepsy and semi-consciousness in a diabetic.

There are, however, many other types of serious illness which can just as often start at work as anywhere else. The capacity to recognise serious illness with certainty comes with experience. The only reliable working rule is: **if in doubt, always play safe and send for help, or refer to a trained doctor or nurse**. The seriously ill patient should be kept lying down until expert help arrives.

In reaching a decision, the first aider will find it helpful to ask the following questions:

- Is the patient able or unable to do his job?
- Does the patient *look* ill?
- Is the patient's colour different from what it usually is?
- Does the patient stand or sit as though in pain?
- Is there any sweating?
- Is breathing laboured or rapid?
- Does the patient complain of pain on breathing? Is the patient feeling sick?

- Has he or she vomited or had diarrhoea?
- Is any pain the patient may complain of unusual for him or her?

Only when the first aider is satisfied that the condition is indeed trivial is he justified in proceeding further on his own.

Care of minor aches and pains

First aiders may only give medicaments if authorised to do so by a doctor or trained occupational health nurse. This is the official guideline and like all such doctrines it should be interpreted with common sense. It is always better not to give medicaments until an expert has had the opportunity to make a diagnosis or at least exclude serious disease.

Using a thermometer

It is as well for every first aider to know how to take a patient's temperature and read a clinical thermometer. It has been a surprise to

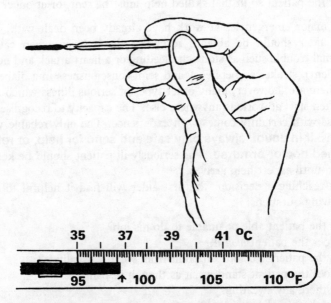

Figure 13.1   Reading a clinical thermometer. This may have a spherical or oblong mercury container and is held in the right hand and slowly rotated until the mercury in the stem is seen magnified. When the thermometer is in the correct position the two parallel lines just below the '90' or '35' act as a guide to finding the mercury

discover how many first aiders cannot carry out these simple tasks. Here an ounce of demonstration is worth a pound of precept.

1   The thermometer should be held in the right hand and slowly rotated (*see* Fig. 13.1). At a certain point, it will be seen that its contents are magnified, and the column of mercury which it contains shows up quite clearly. An arrow or other special mark indicates the *normal* figure of 98.4 degrees Fahrenheit or 37° Centigrade. The mercury column should be well below this.

2   If the mercury column is above, up to, or even near the normal mark, the thermometer should be shaken vigorously until the mercury is well down in the lower nineties.

3   The thermometer is placed in the patient's mouth, under the tongue, and the mouth must be kept shut. It must remain in place for at least two full minutes; this applies to the so-called *half-minute* thermometer as well as to the *two-minute* one. The mark to which the mercury has risen indicates the patient's temperature.

4   Before the thermometer is replaced in its case, it should be carefully washed under a cold tap, dried with a piece of clean cotton wool strip and shaken down. If washed under a hot tap, the mercury may expand so much that it breaks the thermometer.

The first aider may legitimately take the temperature of any patient who 'feels ill'. If the temperature is above normal, the patient must be referred to a trained nurse or doctor. However, a normal or subnormal temperature does not necessarily mean that there is nothing the matter. If the patient looks or seems in any way ill, referral is essential.

Taking a pulse

Taking the pulse at the wrist is more difficult than taking a temperature. It is outside the scope of the average first aider, but pulse-taking techniques may profitably be taught in advanced first aid courses. (*See* also page 51.)

Administering mild medicaments

When the first aider works under the supervision of a nurse, he or she will decide what medicaments, especially analgesics, can be given, and when. In the Harlow Industrial Health Service the following have been authorised.

Compound magnesium trisilicate powder
(Dose; one to two teaspoonfuls in water.) This may be safely and

beneficially given to the patient with a hangover, or to the regular gastric sufferer who is under medical treatment but is caught without his or her own medicine. They should not be given to anyone who appears to be ill. Unless the mixture gives speedy relief the patient should be referred. Severe stomach pain should never be treated by the first aider.

Aspirin or paracetamol tablets
(Dose 1–2 tablets.) These relieve the ordinary headaches, and may help women workers who have pain during periods. It is wise for period pain to be dealt with only by women first aiders. A severe headache, or a headache accompanied by any other symptoms, should always be referred to a trained nurse or doctor. Some people are sensitive to aspirin, or have been advised not to take it. Always check on this before you give a patient aspirin.

Throat tablets
These give some relief for coughs and colds. Most tablets can be sucked once an hour, up to four tablets in all. In such cases the temperature should be taken if the patient looks at all ill. Sore throats are best referred, as also are coughs or colds accompanied by pain in the chest.

Chest pain

All chest pain must be treated seriously and referred to a nurse or doctor for diagnosis. Severe chest pains, if due to a heart attack, will cause shock. The treatment is exactly the same as for any case of shock except that the patient should sit up rather than lie down (*see* page 56). The carotid pulse will not necessarily be fast and weak, but the patient will be anxious, have a poor colour, and may feel cold and clammy. Reassurance is essential and help must be called at once – a doctor or nurse, and an ambulance.

Abdominal pain

Mild indigestion is relatively common and will always respond to antacids, as described above (magnesium trisilicate), and often to a drink of milk. However the first aider should not attempt to make a diagnosis and should only treat a patient with abdominal pain within the guidelines laid down by a nurse or doctor.

When pain is severe the patient must be treated for shock and help obtained immediately, if necessary by calling an ambulance. Nothing should be given by mouth.

Review questions

1 What are the rules about giving medicines to patients?
2 A man complains of 'indigestion' and holds the front of his chest. What do you do?

14   Moving patients

As a general rule, any severely injured or ill person should be moved as little as possible until experienced ambulance workers, nurses or a doctor are available. The transport of the injured is a specialised branch of first aid, calling for considerable practical training and experience. Such training and experience is possessed by ambulance workers, and is rightly emphasised in the St John courses. The industrial first aider may occasionally have to move someone out of a position of immediate and continuing danger, and in emergency may have to undertake a longer carry to an ambulance or first aid post. To meet these emergencies, some practical experience, on the lines set out below, is essential. For the demonstrations of work here described the only equipment needed is:

- a stretcher;
- two blankets;
- a strong scarf.

It is difficult but not impossible to move an injured person safely without a stretcher. It is easier both to load and to carry a stretcher with four bearers than with two. It is easier to move a patient without a stretcher with two bearers than with one. But in emergency one person can move another provided that the proper techniques have been learnt.

Preparing a stretcher

If two blankets are available, they should be arranged on the stretcher in what is known as the *fishtail* position (*see* Fig. 14.1). The patient's feet and legs are covered with the *fishtail* and the body and head are wrapped in the lower blanket, tucking in firmly with the longer side (*see* Fig. 14.2).

If only one blanket is available, it should be arranged on the stretcher diagonally. The patient is then folded into the blanket, with the longer angle turned over on top and tucked in (*see* Fig. 14.3).

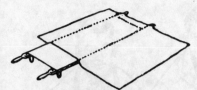 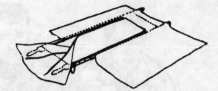

Figure 14.1 Preparing a stretcher using two blankets – the *fishtail* method. Note that there is more of the first blanket on the one side of the stretcher than on the other, and that there will be four thicknesses of blanket under the patient's body, but only one thickness under the head

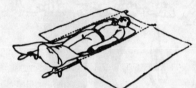 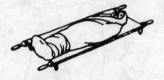

Figure 14.2 The *fishtail* method with the patient in position. The feet are tucked up in the fishtail and the body and head wrapped in the lower blanket, using the longer side for the final tuck-in

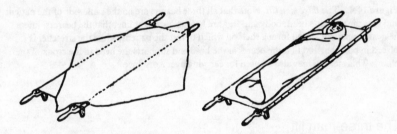

Figure 14.3 Using a single blanket on a stretcher to its best advantage. The blanket is placed diagonally with more on one side than the other. The larger section will be used for the final tuck-in

Loading a stretcher

Ideally, there should be four loaders, one of whom must give orders so that all act together. Three loaders lift the patient; the fourth pushes the stretcher, with blanket or blankets, under the lifted patient, so that he or she can be gently lowered in the right position on the stretcher.

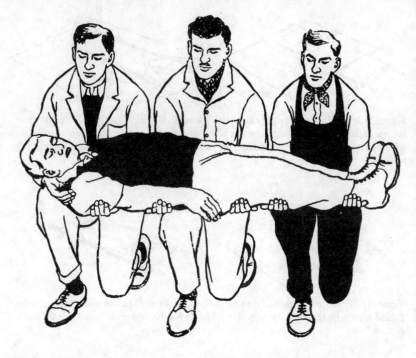

Figure 14.4   The *three man lift*. Note that all three bearers are on the same side of the patient and that the patient's head, body and legs are kept in a straight line, that the bearers' knees nearest the patient's head form a shelf on which to rest the patient, while the stretcher is placed in position, and that the bearer at the head end supports the head in the crook of the elbow. This method may also be used for carrying over a distance

The three-man lift

The *three-man lift* (*see* Fig. 14.4.) is an art to be perfected by practice. Its object is to lift the patient while keeping the head, body and legs in a straight line.

1   All three helpers must be on the *same* side of the patient.
2   They all kneel on one knee, in each case the knee nearer the patient's feet. Their other knees – the knees nearer the patient's head – form a shelf on which the patient can be rested.
3   Hands and arms are gently but firmly insinuated right under the patient.
4   The first helper raises the head and shoulders. The second, who should be the strongest, raises the chest and abdomen. The third raises

the legs, with one arm under the thighs and the other under the calves, taking care not to let the feet sag and the knees bend.

5 When all are ready, the leader gives the command to lift, and the patient is raised and rested on the lifters' bent knees, so that the stretcher can be slipped into position.

6 The leader must give the command to lower, so that all three moves as one.

The three-man lift may also be used for carrying a patient a short distance. It is then spoken of as the *human stretcher*. If only three loaders are available, they will use the three-man lift and carry the patient to the stretcher.

The straddle walk

If there are only two loaders available, both should stand astride the patient, facing his or her head. The first passes the arms under the patient's shoulders; the second passes one arm under the buttocks and the other under the calves. When both are in position, the loader in the rear gives the command to lift. With short steps, they then walk *over* the stretcher, and lower the patient on to it. This procedure is known as the *straddle walk* (*see* Fig. 14.5).

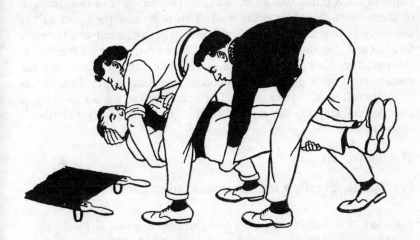

Figure 14.5 The *two man lift* or *straddle walk*. Both bearers stand aside the patient, facing his or her head. That first passes the arms under the patient's shoulders; the second passes one arm under the buttocks and the other under the calves. The bearer in the rear gives commands

Loading an unconscious patient

It is sometimes necessary to load an unconscious patient on to a stretcher. The rules are these:

- *lift* in the prone position;
- *carry* in the semi-prone position.

Attempts to lift in the semi-prone position are dangerous, as the unconscious patient may roll out of the lifters' arms. Carriage in the prone position is difficult because of the position of the patient's arms; also the airway may be obstructed.

The transport of the patient with a broken back or neck has already been dealt with under the care of fractures in Chapter 7 (*see* page 77).

Carrying a stretcher

Carrying a stretcher is more difficult than it looks. Practical experience is needed both as a bearer and as a 'patient'. It is surprisingly easy for the unskilled to tip a patient off a stretcher.

There has been much discussion as to whether it is better to carry a patient head first or feet first. We support the conventional St John method of carrying feet first, though there are exceptions to this, for example when lifting into an ambulance. The strongest or two strongest of the carriers should be at the head. This is because the upper half of the body is heavier than the lower half. The command to lift, move forward and stop should be given by one of the carriers at the rear end of the stretcher. Care must be taken to keep the stretcher level, and the bearers must walk out of the traditional marching step; otherwise the stretcher will soon start to swing. The smoothest carry is achieved by all four bearers adopting the rhythm: 'inner foot – outer foot; inner foot – outer foot' etc.

The blanket lift

Four people can carry a severely injured patient using a single blanket.

Figure 14.6   The blanket lift: (top) to get the blanket under the patient three bearers pull the patient towards them, while a fourth inserts the rolled blanket under the patient; (middle) the patient is lowered on to the roll, the bearers move over to the other side of the patient and again pull the patient towards them, the fourth bearer pulls out the rolled blanket; (bottom) the blanket on either side of the patient is rolled and one bearer takes hold of each half roll. Considerable tension is needed to keep the blanket lift

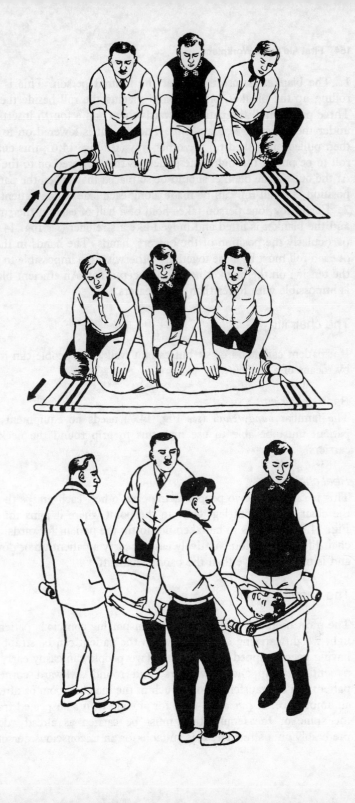

1   The blanket is inserted under the injured person. This is done by rolling up the blanket longways and placing the roll beside the patient. Three people pull the patient towards them and a fourth inserts the roll under the patient (*see* Fig. 14.6). The patient is lowered on to the roll, then pulled or pushed up the other way (*see* Fig. 14.6); this enables the roll to be pulled through. The patient is then lowered on to the blanket. At the outset, the blanket should be so placed that, when the patient is in position, a small roll can be made along each side of the patient.

2   For lifting, one person takes hold of a half of each of the small rolls, and the blanket is lifted and moved like a stretcher (*see* Fig. 14.6). Note particularly the position of the bearers' hands. The hands in the middle of each roll must be close together. Otherwise it is impossible to maintain the tension on the blanket needed to keep it flat. An efficient blanket lift is impossible with fewer than four bearers.

The chair lift

If a patient can stand or sit but cannot walk, two people can move him by means of a *chair lift*.

Bandy chair lift
The familiar *bandy chair* (*see* Fig. 14.7) needs no equipment, but the patient must be able to use his arms to grip round the necks of the carriers.

Real chair lift
This is carried by two people facing each other: each grasps the back of the chair and a front leg, close to the point where it joins the seat (*see* Fig. 14.8). Care has to be taken not to tip the patient forwards. The real chair lift makes it comparatively easy to carry a patient up or down stairs and is more effective than the bandy chair lift.

The carrying chair

The most useful all-purpose aid to transporting conscious patients is the light-weight carrying chair into which the patient can be strapped, after having been wrapped in a blanket. Two people can easily carry a heavy patient both up and downstairs, and round awkward corners. The patient can be transferred to a couch in the medical room or directly into an ambulance. It *cannot* be used for anyone with a suspected fracture of the spine or the femur; they must be carried as already described, preferably on a stretcher. It is suitable for an unconscious person only if

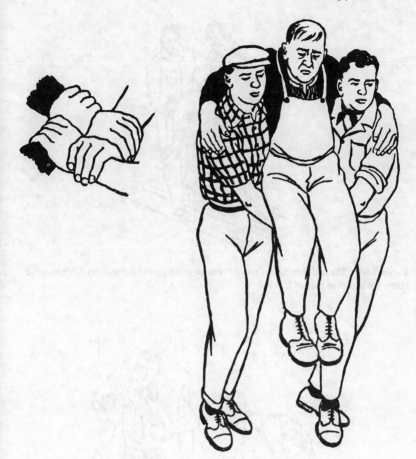

Figure 14.7   The *bandy chair lift*. The patient must be able to use his or her arms to grip around the neck of the carriers

the patient is very carefully supervised all the time to ensure that the airway is clear, and if the patient is transferred into the recovery position as soon as possible.

Single-handed lifts

The pick-a-back

If a patient can just stand and has the use of the arms, the familiar *pick-a-back* is useful. For the pick-a-back, the carrier must use both his hands and cannot therefore climb a ladder.

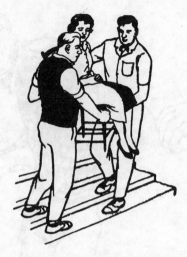

Figure 14.8   The *real chair lift*: of special value in going up and down stairs. Care must be taken not to tilt the patient forward

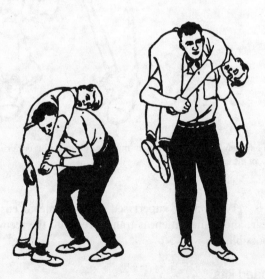

Figure 14.9   The *fireman's lift*: (left) the rescuer grasps the patient's right wrist with the left hand; the rescuer's right shoulder goes into the patient's stomach; the right arm is between the patient's legs and the right hand grasps the patient's right leg; (right) the weight of the patient is taken on the rescuer's right shoulder; the patient's right arm is pulled well over the rescuer's left shoulder; the patient's right wrist is grasped by the rescuer's right hand, leaving the left hand free

The fireman's lift

The *fireman's lift* leaves a hand free, and so makes ladder-climbing possible. It demands considerable strength on the part of the carrier, and a good balance; it cannot therefore be used if the patient is very heavy, unless the carrier is proportionately strong.

The patient must be able to stand upright, facing the carrier. The carrier grasps the patient's right wrist with the left hand, then bends down until the head is just under the patient's right hand. This brings the carrier's right shoulder level with the lower part of the patient's abdomen. The right arm is then placed between (or round) the patient's legs, and the leg or legs are grasped firmly. The weight of the patient is then taken on his right shoulder. As the carrier rises to stand upright, the patient is pulled across both shoulders. The patient's right wrist is then transferred to the rescuer's right hand, thus leaving the left hand free. (*See* Fig. 14.9.)

A little practice will soon demonstrate the value and the limitations of the fireman's lift.

The neck drag

The single-handed movement and rescue of an unconscious or badly injured patient is effected by the *neck-drag*. The only equipment needed is a strong scarf, belt or tie. The patient's wrists are tied together. The rescuer kneels astride the patient, with his or her knees in the patient's armpits. The rescuer loops the patient's hands over his or her own neck

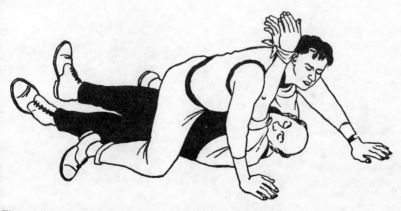

Figure 14.10   The *neckdrag*: the patient's wrists are tied together and looped over the rescuer's neck

(*see* Fig. 14.10). As the rescuer crawls forwards, the patient is pulled forward on the rescuer's own neck and shoulders.

If a patient has to be pulled a short distance only, he or she may instead be grasped under the shoulders and pulled along head-and-shoulders first in a semi-sitting position. On no account must a patient be dragged by the feet, as the risk of injury to the head is then great.

Review questions

1   How would you lift a patient who had fallen downstairs and was unconscious? (There is a fire and you have to move him.)
2   When is a carrying chair not suitable? Why not?

15 Training first aiders

Teaching first aid

This book is intended to offer both those who learn and those who teach first aid a sound basis for study. The teacher who accompanies careful study of each chapter with practical demonstrations and frequent practice in the classroom will equip new first aiders with both the knowledge and the experience necessary to cope well with accidents and emergencies at work and the day-to-day running of the first aid post.

Good first aid teaching is an art which can be learnt only by practice and by trial and error. The teacher who talks too much is usually less effective than the teacher who says too little. The class must be encouraged to participate but not allowed to get out of hand. The exhibitionist must be firmly shut up and the shy ones allowed to have their say. Above all, the class must **do things for themselves**.

In all teaching, repetition is of immense importance. The advice of the wise old lay preacher may be recalled: "First, I tells 'em what I'm going to say. Then I says it. Then I tells 'em what I've said." Throughout, there is some *deliberate* repetition. It is part of the teaching process.

As we stated in Chapter 1 of the book the qualities a good first aid teacher must look for and encourage in his or her students are that they are:

- careful in their observations;
- accurate in their interrogation;
- honest in their judgment;
- ready to admit mistakes and learn from experience;
- clean, systematic and gentle in their treatment of patients;
- quiet, unanxious and unhurried in manner.

Planning a course

Provided the lecturer is concise and avoids irrelevance and discursiveness, the course, as set out here, can be covered comfortably in six lecture-demonstrations, each lasting 60–75 minutes. A fully stocked first aid box and a blackboard must be available for each lecture-demonstration. It is an advantage not to try to cover the course in less than six weeks. This gives class members, who are inevitably busy people, an opportunity to read over and think about what they have learnt.

The teacher should prepare detailed lecture notes before each class, and revise them each time a lecture is repeated.

Points to remember in preparing lectures

1　Both doctors and nurses, when teaching, have to shake themselves free from the way they were taught as students. Unnecessary technical terms and theoretical knowledge must be jetisoned. Simplicity is all important.

2　Today, technical knowledge and ability in scientific subjects has become an everyday requirement in industry and commerce. Professional workers and skilled technicians will be quick to criticise faulty reasoning behind any procedure. Vague and imprecise talk of *germs* and *antiseptics* by the teacher will be quickly detected and queried.

3　First aiders must think for themselves, but they are not required to make precise diagnoses. They need to know how to decide quickly whether a particular illness and injury is within their power to treat. They will do this better if they are not confused by medical inessentials.

4　A number of time-honoured first aid treatments are unnecessarily complicated and of doubtful value. These are best left out – they have not been included in this book.

5　Practical medicine is built on the hypothesis of *calculated risk*. Quite unconsciously, the doctor in daily practice is continually making use of the theory of probabilities. The doctor decides on the probable diagnosis and acts accordingly. If doctors set out to exclude every improbability, they would block the hospital machine, and patients might die in the interim. First aid must be taught and conducted on the same basis. The first aider must be sure of the correct way of dealing with the common injuries. The same way may not be quite right for the rare complicated contingency. But it is better to accept this slight risk than to burden the first aider with complications who then becomes confused when facing the common situation.

An outline for the course is suggested below.

Lecture 1   The nature of industrial first aid; the first aider's tools and responsibilities

How industrial first aid resembles and differs from ordinary first aid; the first aid box and where to put it; the contents of the box; individual sterilised dressings; cotton wool; adhesive plaster; protection from oil; the roller bandage; the triangular bandage; other items; what to leave out; record keeping; notification of accidents; responsibilities of the first aider; prevention of AIDS and Hepatitis B.

Lecture 2   Wounds and wound treatment

Major and minor wounds; bleeding; infection; general treatment; foreign bodies; grazes and crushes; wounds of the chest and abdomen; nose bleeding; ruptured varicose vein; contusions; blisters; insect bites and stings.

Lecture 3   Shock and other effects of serious injury; fractures, strains and sprains

Shock; what the shocked patient looks like; what happens in shock; results of fluid loss; management of shock; crush injuries; fainting.

General consideration of fractures; bones commonly broken and how to recognise them; first aid care of fractures, general and particular; strains and sprains; dislocations.

Lecture 4   Burns and scalds; physical and chemical injuries

Minor and serious burns; different kinds of burn; objects of first aid; treatment of trivial, medium and serious burns; rescue from burning buildings.

Electric burns; electric shock, types, symptoms and treatment. Heat injuries; types, care and prevention.

Chemical injuries; acids, quick and slow acting; alkalis; chemical skin irritation; chemical poisons.

Notifiable diseases. Role of the DHSS.

The Health and Safety at Work Act.

Lecture 5   Unconsciousness; gassing and asphyxia; artificial respiration

Unconsciousness where the cause is obvious; where the cause is probable; with no obvious cause; care of the unconscious patient; internal causes of unconsciousness; fainting, fits, strokes, diabetes, alcohol, hysteria.

Rescue of a gas casualty; industrial gases; irritants; smothering gases; tissue poisons; narcotising gases; treatment of a gas casualty; dust and fumes.

Artificial respiration; when it is needed; speed; preliminaries; the mouth-to-mouth method; the airway; the Holger Neilsen method; resuscitators; oxygen; the airway.

Lecture 6   The eye; minor ailments; transport

Importance of eye injuries; examining an eye; removal of a foreign body; glass; scratches; dust; foreign body within the globe of the eye; welding and the eye; chemical splashes; bandaging an eye; prevention of eye injury.

Aches and pains; reading a thermometer; tablets.

Moving an injured person; preparing a stretcher; the three-man lift; carrying a stretcher; the blanket lift; the chair-lift; single-handed lifts; the neck-drag.

Practical work

It is essential to spend an adequate amount of time on practical work. This can be done at the end of each session. In particular, sufficient time must be allowed for each student to practise artificial respiration.

Examinations in first aid

How should examinations in occupational first aid be conducted?
The purpose of the examination must always be kept in mind. It is to see if the candidate is capable of doing first aid work safely and efficiently. If the first aider can do the job, he or she should pass. If not, it is in the interest of all that the candidate should fail. We find that the great majority of candidates who have conscientiously attended a course based on the teaching set out here will in fact pass. If a candidate passes but is found to have inadequate knowledge of one subject he or she should be told this and re-examined in this subject later.

In our experience group examinations are useless. Each candidate must be examined orally, and must also do certain simple practical tests. At work the first aider will do most of the work and make most decisions alone, so his or her individual capacity without the support of colleagues must be assessed. It is required that all first aid examinations are held by two independent examiners – say, a nursing sister and a doctor. They should ask alternate questions but both should score all answers. We mark each answer from 0–5. A fully-stocked first aid box should be at hand and open. One of the examiners should allow himself or herself to be used as a subject. In a fifteen minute oral examination it is usually possible to get through eight to ten questions.

Is it right to let first aiders know the kind of questions they may be asked at examination?

This problem arises in every type of examination. The short answer is that, regardless of whether it is right or wrong, resourceful candidates are bound to find out the questions asked previously from those who have taken the examination before. So for most examinations, the questions previously asked are now published for candidates to study.

Knowing the type of question likely to be asked has one real advantage. It takes away some of the anxiety with which the candidate approaches the examination and enables him to do more justice to himself. Moreover, the study of a well-selected group of questions is an excellent method of revision.

What type of questions may be asked?

Questions should be practical rather than theoretical and related as far as possible to the kind of situations which the first aider will meet at work. It is important to achieve a good scatter, so that ignorance in any particular field does not go undetected. Accordingly, the following specimen questions are arranged under eight subject headings. At least one question should be asked on each of these subjects:

- Wounds
- Severe injury
- Fractures
- Burns and chemical injuries
- The unconscious patient
- Artificial respiration
- Electric shock
- The eye
- Moving a patient

Wounds
1 I have a two-inch long cut on my forearm which is bleeding rather

badly. Select from the first aid box the dressing to apply, and show me how you would apply it.

2   Quite quickly blood comes through the dressing you have just applied. What would you do to the wound, the arm, and to the patient generally?

3   I have a small cut on my finger. How would you decide whether to deal with it yourself or to send it on to someone else?

   If you decided to deal with it yourself, how would you clean and dress it?

4   The patient has to return to an oily job. How would you protect the wound and the dressing you have applied?

5   A man wearing rubber-soled shoes has trod on a nail projecting from a plank. What would you do?

6   A middle-aged woman wheeling a tea trolley has slipped and cut her leg on a steel bar. The cut although small is pouring out blood. What has happened? How would you treat her?

7   Blood is squirting out from a cut on the wrist. How would you deal with this?

8   How would you treat a blister on, say, the heel?

Severe injury

9   A patient has collapsed in the lavatory. He is just conscious, pale, and sweating. His skin feels cold. What is his condition called? What has probably caused it? How could you look after him?

10   You are called to a man with a severe crush injury of the hand. Describe his general condition. How would you look after him? He says he feels thirsty. Would you give him anything to drink? Why, or why not?

Fractures

11   What is meant by the word fracture? How can you tell if a patient has got a fracture? Suppose I had got a fracture of my forearm, how would you deal with it?

12   What does a patient with a fractured hip look like? And a fractured wrist? And what does a patient with a fractured rib complain of?

13   Show me how you would use a triangular bandage as sling.

Burns and chemical injuries

14 I have a small burn on my finger from a soldering iron. Show me how you would treat it.

15 How would you deal with a petrol burn involving, say, six square inches on the arm?

16 How would you set about rescuing someone from a burning building?

17 I am pouring some acid from a carboy and some spills over my arm and hand, and on to my trousers. How would you deal with the situation? Suppose it had been caustic soda. What would you do then?

18 How would you deal with a chemical splash in the eye?

19 How would you deal with cement or lime in the eye?

20 Tell me the names of some substances which are used in industry and may cause dermatitis. What would you do if a worker came to you with a complaint of skin irritation?

The unconscious patient

21 You are called to an elderly man who is lying on his back unconscious and breathing heavily. What would you suspect was the matter with him? What would you do?

22 What would you do for a patient who is having an epileptic fit?

23 What are the recovery and the prone positions? When do you make use of these positions?

24 An unconscious patient smells of alcohol. What conclusion would you draw?

25 A fellow-worker whom you know to have diabetes comes up to you and tells you rather aggressively that he is feeling muzzy and can see double. What would you do for him? Why?

26 How would you set about rescuing someone who has been overcome by coal gas?

Electric shock

27 How would you deal with a case of electric shock?

28 Is there anything peculiar about electric burns? What do they look like and how would you deal with them?

29   In what position would you place a patient before starting artificial respiration? What would be your position? Describe the movements you would make and the rhythm. What apparatus might help you?

The eye
30   A patient says he has got something in his eye. Show me how you would examine him.

31   You can see a foreign body on the white of the eye. What would you do?

  Suppose you have to send the patient on for expert help, what would you do first?

32   The patient says he was using a hammer and chisel when he got something in his eye. On examination you can see nothing unusual. What conclusion would you draw and what steps would you take?

Miscellaneous
33   Can you read a clinical thermometer? What is the reading on this one?

34   In our first aid box, there are three kinds of tablet. What are they and what are they used for? What is the dose of each of them?

35   Three of you have put a patient on to a stretcher. Where would you stand? How would you do the job?

36   If four of you lift someone and you had only a blanket available, how would you set about it?

37   If you were single-handed, how would you move an unconscious patient out of danger?

Having attended a course and passed an examination in industrial first aid, will the first aider receive a certificate?
A first aider should certainly receive a certificate. The certificate issued by the Harlow Industrial Health Service to its trained first aiders is shown in Fig. 15.1. Any first aid course and certificate have to be approved by the Chief Inspector of Factories. Such a certificate is valid for three years. Thereafter, the first aider must attend a refresher course and obtain a fresh certificate of competence.

Official approval of courses based on this book

Arrangements have been made for firms anywhere in Britain to affiliate

HARLOW   **INDUSTRIAL**

HEALTH   **SERVICE**

Edinburgh House
Templefields Harlow

Industrial First Aid Certificate

This is to certify that

----

has attended a course of lecture-demonstrations
on Industrial First Aid, and has passed an oral
and practical examination to the satisfaction of
the Service

Date _____   _____

              Chairman of the Council
              of the Service

              Medical Director

Figure 15.1 A specimen first aid cerificate

to the Harlow Industrial Health Service for the purpose of giving first aid training courses based on this book.

The Health and Safety Executive, under the 1981 Regulations, has recognised the service as an *approved training organisation*.

With the approval of the HSE, firms or groups of firms with their own medical officer can affiliate to the Harlow Industrial Health Service for first aid training. Certificates to candidates who have reached the required standard are issued by the Service, and these fulfil the requirements of the regulations.

Full details of the arrangements and the conditions for affiliation can be obtained from:

The Medical Director,
Harlow Industrial Health Service,
Edinburgh Way,
Harlow,
Essex.

Any firm or group of firms with their own doctor or suitably qualified nurse can apply direct to the Health and Safety Executive for recognition as a training organization in its own right. Organizers will have to provide details of the course they propose to run and of the qualifications of the lecturers and examiners. When approved, every first aid course must be notified to the local employment nursing advisor in advance. The advisor may wish to attend and will wish to ensure that standards of teaching are being maintained.

Who can practise occupational first aid?

The official code of practice specifies three kinds of persons to be involved in the provision of first aid. These are as follows.

(a) An *appointed person* is a person provided by the employer to take charge of the situation, e.g. to call an ambulance, if a serious injury, accident or major illness occurs and there is no first aider available. The appointed person will also take charge of the first aid equipment. No training is required for appointed persons, although knowledge of simple first aid procedures outlined above is highly desirable. However, such persons should be appointed in writing by the employer, and their names brought to the attention of all employees.

(b) A *first aider* is a person who has been trained and holds a current first aid certificate. The training requirements for first aiders are given below.

(c) An *occupational first aider* is a person who has been trained and holds a current occupational first aid certificate, and who has received specialised instruction concerning the particular first aid requirements of his employer's undertaking. The training requirements for occupational first aiders are outlined below.

For the purpose of the approved code, the training and qualifications of medical practitioners and state registered, registered general, state enrolled and enrolled nurses count as qualifications for first aiders or occupational first aiders.

We are by no means certain that the use of the *appointed person* (*see* (a) above) as an untrained first aider is in the interest of a company or of first aid. We would recommend that only those with knowledge of and training in first aid be given first aid responsibilities.

What are the official first aid requirements?

The guidance notes associated with the approved code outline the subjects that should be included in a training course for first aiders. These are:

(a) resuscitation;
(b) control of bleeding;
(c) treatment of shock;
(d) treatment of the unconscious patient;
(e) dressing and immobilisation of injured parts;
(f) the contents of first aid boxes and their use;
(g) transport of sick and injured patients;
(h) recognition of illness;
(i) treatment of injuries;
(j) treatment of burns and scalds;
(k) simple record keeping;
(l) poisons and substances capable of causing poisoning;
(m) personal hygiene in dealing with wounds; *and*;
(n) communication and delegation in an emergency.

The official duration of a course, including examination, should normally be at least 4 days. The examination should cover both theory and practice, and every trainee should be required to demonstrate proficiency in resuscitation, control of bleeding and treatment of the unconscious patient.

Certificates of qualification in first aid are valid for 3 years only. A refresher course, followed by re-examination, is required before re-certification.

Occupational first aiders should have completed training in the subjects listed above for the first aider's training course. In addition, the following should be included:

(a) safety and hygiene in treating the patient;

(b) detailed record keeping;

(c) detailed training on particular aspects of first aid relevant to the undertaking, e.g. treatment of eye injuries, rescue techniques, use of protective equipment and emergency procedures; and

(d) chemical hazards and their treatment specific to the place of work, e.g. use of cyanide, platinum salts, acids and alkalis.

All such training must be undertaken by an organisation approved by the Health and Safety Executive under the Regulations (*see* also Chapter 16).

Further reading

What other books are of value to the factory first aider who is keenly interested in first aid?

Health in Industry by Dr Donald Hunter of the London Hospital (Pelican Books) is a fascinating account of all aspects of industrial disease and its prevention. Though technical, it is easy to read. However, some excellent practical first aiders may find the science beyond their comprehension.

Health in Industry by Professor R. C. Browne of Newcastle (Arnold) is the best available simple book on the working environment in relation to health, accidents and disease.

Health and Safety Practice by Jeremy Stranks and Malcolm Dewis (Pitman) is a RoSPA publication providing a comprehensive and up-to-date introduction to the practice of health and safety at work.

First Aid Manual, the authorised manual of the St John Ambulance Association, the St Andrew's Ambulance Association and the British Red Cross Society, is now the standard text-book of the three national first aid teaching organisations. It has recently been completely revised and rewritten, and on most subjects its teaching is now completely in line with ours. Its only disadvantage is that it covers so much that the learner may become confused. Nevertheless, every intelligent first aider will find it an invaluable work of reference.

Fundamentals of First Aid by Dr R. A. Mustard, the official publication of the St John Ambulance of Canada, covers much of the ground dealt with in this book. It represents an original approach to the teaching of first aid. It is, however, hard to obtain in this country.

First Aid in Coal Mines, another St John publication, prepared in association with the Medical Service of British Coal is a clinical work of outstanding value. Apart from the specialised audience for whom it is planned, it will be of help to all first aid workers in heavy industry.

The First Aid Civil Defence Handbook No. 6 (HMSO) is a comprehensive training manual for civil defence workers.

Artificial Respiration by Dr T O Garland (Faber and Faber) is a beautifully illustrated little classic. It should be read by every enthusiastic first aider and by every teacher of first aid. It was written before mouth-to-mouth respiration was introduced.

Resuscitation of the Unconscious Victim by Dr Peter Safar and M C McMahon (C C Thomas, Springfield, Illinois) gives a detailed account of mouth-to-mouth artificial respiration.

The Health and Safety Commission

The Health and Safety Commission publishes a wide range of information sheets and *Guidance Notes* on most common health hazards at work, as well as a bimonthly *Newsletter*. *Guidance Notes* cost between one and four pounds, leaflets and posters are free. The complete list of available publications can be obtained from the following addresses:

The Health and Safety Executive:

Broad Lane,	Baynards House,	St Hugh's House,
Sheffield	1 Chepstow Place,	Stanley Precinct,
S3 7HQ	London	Bootle,
Tel: 0742-752539	W2 4TF	Merseyside, L20 3QY
	Tel: 01-221 0416 *or*	Tel: 051-951 4381
	01-221 0870	

A display card on mouth-to-mouth resuscitation (size: 22 in × 13½ in) can be obtained from:

Ernest Benn Ltd,
Bouverie House,
Fleet Street,
London EC4

The official booklet

Everyone who is organising first aid arrangements for an occupational health service, or is conducting a course on first aid at work should obtain a copy of this official booklet. It is entitled:
First Aid at Work, Health and Safety series booklet HS (R) 11, HMSO (ISBN 0-11-883446).

It covers the following matters:

- The Health and Safety (First Aid) Regulations, approved in 1981, which came into force on 1 July, 1982.
- The approved Code of Practice based on the Regulations.
- Guidance Notes expanding the Approved Code of Practice. These Guidance Notes deal, among other things, with the following:

(a) equipment and facilities: first aid boxes, first aid rooms, protective clothing;
(b) suitable persons for training;
(c) liaison with local ambulance service;
(d) record keeping;
(e) training – instruction, refresher courses, instructors;
(f) special needs of small establishments;
(g) guidance for employers;
(h) brief general first aid guidance for insertion in first aid boxes.

Film strips

Well prepared film strips are useful adjuncts to first aid teaching, particularly in refresher courses. As teaching aids, we have found them more valuable than cinematograph films, as they usually cover more ground and also enable the teacher to participate in the process of teaching. The accompanying lecture notes must be very carefully studied and adjusted as necessary to meet the needs of the audience before the film strip is shown.

Films

There are many films available demonstrating resuscitation techniques, for purchase and hire.
Recommended are those product by:
Laerdal Medical Ltd
Laerdal House
Goodmead Road, Orpington. Kent. BR6 OHX
Tel: 0689 76634

Teaching aids

Resusci Anne, in many forms, can be purchased from Laerdal Medical Ltd, as can wall posters and flip charts. A manikin, whether full-size or torso only, is invaluable for practising artificial respiration and cardio-pulmonary resuscitation. (*See also* page 118).

16 The legal framework

The Health and Safety at Work Act, 1974

The Health and Safety at Work Act was passed in 1974 and resulted in a reorganization of the Government departments responsible for inspecting and advising all workplaces on occupational health and safety.

A central, independent *Health and Safety Commission* is responsible for setting standards, drawing up regulations and Codes of good practice, and, through their officers in the *Health and Safety Executive*, they employ Inspectors to ensure that the regulations are followed. The Executive (HSE) employs doctors and nurses in an *Employment Medical Advisory Service*. The functions of this service are:-

- To advise employers, unions and doctors in other specialties, on health problems at work.
- On request, a doctor or nurse will visit any firm to advise on any health hazard, either in general or on behalf of any individual.
- Medical or other examinations may be required by regulation when employees are working in jobs known to be hazardous. These are often delegated to the firm's own doctor.

Inspectors, doctors and nurses all work on an area basis from a local office where they can be contacted. The address of any local office can be obtained by writing or telephoning:
Public Enquiry Point,
Baynards House,
1 Chepstow Place,
London
W2 4TF.
Tel: 01–221–0416 *or* 01–221 0870.

The *Environmental Health Inspectors* of the local authority are responsible for inspecting many non-industrial firms, such as shops and offices. They are also responsible for checking canteens and ensuring that food is hygienically prepared. They have to be notified if there are any cases of suspected food poisoning.

New regulations covering first aid

New government rules covering first aid in all workplaces were introduced in 1981 by the Health and Safety Executive. These rules consist of three parts: regulations, a code of practice, and guidance notes. Organizations wishing to give training in first aid at work must apply to:
The Chief Employment Nursing Adviser,
Health and Safety Executive,
Employment Medical Advisory Service,
25 Chapel Street,
London,
NW1 5DT.

They will have to get approval for the content of their proposed course and the qualifications of those who will be teaching and examining.

The official booklet *First Aid at Work*, (*see* page 171), can be purchased from:
HMSO
49, High Holborn,
London,
WCIV 6HB.

Contents of first aid Boxes

Under the 1981 First Aid Regulations first aid boxes must contain the items set out in Table 2.1. Table 2.2 gives the supplementary contents which we have found essential for efficient first aid at work. Look again at these tables in chapter 2 and at the official statement of contents which begins on page 10.

Notes

(a) For every item, the quantity officially specified is a minimum only.

(b) The recommended supply of assorted *adhesive wound dressings* is, in our experience, too small. These are by far the most frequently used dressings in industrial first aid. These dressings have to be put up in individual sealed packets. This adds to their cost but in typical work conditions it is an advantage.

(c) There is no practical difference between a *sterile covering for serious wounds* and *sterile unmedicated dressings*. It is possible to purchase *sterile wrapped triangular bandages* and these are best for large wound areas when only a covering dressing is required.

(d) No cotton wool is included. We recommend the use of a cotton wool strip dispenser, or sterile cotton wool balls, and extra 15 gm packets of wool for padding splints, etc.

(e) *Roller bandages* used to be a requirement in the larger factory first aid boxes, but are now omitted from the official list. In our experience they are needed as the best means of protecting adhesive wound dressings from oil and dirt. They are therefore retained in our supplement.

(f) *Hibitane* for stock purposes is normally supplied in a five per cent solution. Half an ounce of this in two-and-a-half pints of water (or 20 ml of stock solution in two litres of water) yields at 0.05% solution. Hibitane is not itself a cleansing agent, but as formulated, a detergent is embodied in the solution.

(g) The proprietary *non-inflammable plaster remover* which we recommend is *Zoff*. It is specially useful for removing obstinate oil and dirt from the skin around a wound before applying the dressing. It may be abused by *sniffers* and so must be carefully controlled.

(h) A roll of *adhesive plaster* (1.3 cm wide) is useful for fixing the ends of dressings and bandages.

(i) Every *first aid box* must be plainly marked *First Aid*, in white on a green background, and should also carry the name and location of the first aid worker in charge of it.

(j) There must be at least one first aid box for every 150 employees. If, however, a properly equipped ambulance room is available, the health and safety inspector can give exemption from this requirement.

(k) Any container used to store first aid dressings, e.g. for use with transport vehicles, must protect the contents from damp and dust. They must always be clearly identifiable as first aid containers with a white cross on a green background as well as the label *First Aid*.

First Aid Regulations, 1981 – official statement of contents

1   First aid boxes or similar containers which are to form part of an establishment's permanent first aid provision should contain only the following items:

(a) card giving the general first aid guidance (set out in the Annex to the guidance notes);

(b) individually wrapped sterile adhesive dressings;

(c) sterile eye pads, with attachment (an example of a suitable eye pad currently available would be the Standard Dressing No 16 BPC);

(d) triangular bandages (these should if possible be sterile; if not, sterile coverings appropriate for serious wounds should also be included);

(e) safety pins;

(f) a selection of sterile unmedicated wound dressings, which should include at least the following:

- medium sized sterile unmedicated dressings (approx 10 cm × 8 cm; examples of suitable dressings currently available are the Standard Dressings No 8 and No 13 BPC);
- large sterile unmedicated dressings (approx 13 cm × 9 cm; examples of suitable dressings currently available are the Standard Dressings No 9 and No 14 BPC and the Ambulance Dressing No 1);
- extra large sterile unmedicated dressings (approx 28 cm × 17.5 cm; an example of a suitable dressing currently available would be the Ambulance Dressing No 3).

2 In cases where the *Hydrogen Cyanide (Fumigation of Buildings) Regulations, 1951, the Hydrogen Cyanide (Fumigation of Ships) Regulations, 1951, the Food Hygiene (General) Regulations, 1970, the Food Hygiene (Docks, Carriers, etc) Regulations 1960* and *the Food Hygiene (Markets, Stalls and Delivery Vehicles) Regulations, 1966* apply, the first aid items specified in those regulations are also suitable and should be kept in first aid boxes or similar containers in addition to the items listed above.

3 Soap and water and disposable drying materials, or suitable equivalents, should also be available. Where tap water is not available, sterile water or sterile normal saline, in disposable containers each holding at least 300 ml, should be kept easily accessible, and near to the first aid box, for eye irrigation.

4 Sufficient quantities of each item should always be available in every first aid box or container; at least the numbers of each item shown in the table 2.1 should be provided.

Travelling first aid kits

The contents of small travelling first aid kits (for use) in establishments where there is dispersed working, or by employees working away from their employer's establishment or by self-employed persons) may vary according to need. However, items included should always be among those specified for boxes (*see* Table 2.1). In general, the following items should be sufficient:

(a) 6 individually wrapped sterile adhesive dressings;

(b) one medium sized sterile unmedicated dressing (approx 10 cm × 8 cm; examples of suitable dressings currently available are the Standard Dressings No 8 and No 13 BPC);

(c) one triangular bandage (this should, if possible, be sterile; if not, a sterile covering appropriate for serious wounds should also be included);

(d) 6 safety pins.

Carrying equipment

The approved code states that where first aiders and occupational first aiders are employed in an establishment the employer should provide appropriate carrying equipment for them to use. In addition it is recommended that where such equipment is provided, blankets should be stored alongside the equipment and in such a way as to keep them free from dust and dampness.

Protective clothing and equipment

Protective clothing and equipment should be provided near the first aid materials where there is a possibility that the first aider or occupational first aider might need protection to avoid becoming a casualty himself while administering first aid. Protective clothing and equipment should always be properly stored and checked regularly to ensure that it remains in good condition.

First aid room

A first aid room is needed when there are over 400 employees or when there are special hazards. When the siting of a new first aid room is under consideration it should, where possible, have toilets nearby and any corridors, lifts etc which lead to the first aid room may need to allow access for a stretcher, wheelchair, carrying chair or wheeled carriage.

The possibility of providing some form of emergency lighting may be considered.

First aid room facilities

The following facilities and equipment should be provided in first aid rooms:

    (a) sink with running hot and cold water always available;
    (b) drinking water when not available on tap;
    (c) paper towels;
    (d) smooth topped working surfaces;
    (e) an adequate supply of sterile dressings and other materials for wound treatment.
    (f) clinical thermometer;
    (g) a couch with pillow and blankets frequently cleaned;
    (h) a suitable store for first aid materials;
    (i) soap and nail brush;
    (j) clean garments for use by first aiders and occupational first aiders;
    (k) suitable refuse container.

Where occupational first aiders are employed in an establishment and any special first aid equipment is needed to deal with the particular hazards of their undertaking, this equipment should also normally be stored in the first aid room.

The approved code of practice states that the first aid room should not normally be used for any other purposes than the rendering of first aid. However, in addition to first aid the room may be used for medical examinations.

Official Guidance Notes

The HSE leaflet, *Official Guidance Notes* is reproduced in Fig. 16.1. (It is specifically stated that these can be reproduced without infringing copyright.) A copy of these notes *must* be included in every first aid box.

Notification of accidents at work

(Thus refers to the Reporting of Injuries, Diseases and Dangerous Occurrences at Work Act, 1985.) When an accident at work leads to the

Guidance Notes on First Aid

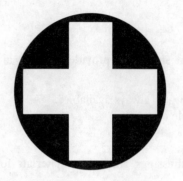

Health and Safety (First-Aid) Regulations 1981

NOTE   *TAKE CARE NOT TO BECOME A CASUALTY YOURSELF WHILE ADMINISTERING FIRST AID. BE SURE TO USE PROTECTIVE CLOTHING AND EQUIPMENT WHERE NECESSARY. IF YOU ARE NOT A TRAINED FIRST-AIDER, SEND IMMEDIATELY FOR THE NEAREST FIRST-AIDER WHERE ONE IS AVAILABLE.*

Advice on treatment

If the assistance of medical or nursing personnel will be required, send for a doctor or nurse (where they are employed at the workplace) or ambulance immediately. When an ambulance is called, arrangements should be made for it to be directed to the scene without delay.

Priorities

(1) *Breathing* If the casualty has stopped breathing, resuscitation must be started at once *before any other treatment is given* and should be continued until breathing is restored or until medical, nursing or ambulance personnel take over.

Mouth-to-mouth resuscitation

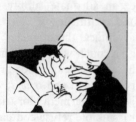

(2) *Bleeding* If bleeding is more than minimal, control it by direct pressure — apply a pad of sterilised dressing or, if necessary direct pressure with fingers or thumb on the bleeding point. Raising a limb if the bleeding is sited there will help reduce the flow of blood (unless the limb is fractured).

(3) *Unconsciousness* Where the patient in unconscious, care must be taken to keep the airway open. This may be done by clearing the mouth and ensuring that the tongue does not block the back of the throat. Where possible, the casualty should be placed in the recovery position.

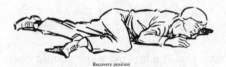

Recovery position

(4) *Broken bones* Unless the casualty is in a position which exposes him to further danger, do not attempt to move a casualty with suspected broken bones or injured joints until the injured parts have been supported. Secure so that the injured parts cannot move.

(5) *Other injuries*

(a) *Burns and scalds* Small burns and scalds should be treated by flushing the affected area with plenty of clean cool water before applying a sterilised dressing or a clean towel. Where the burn is large or deep, simply apply a dry sterile dressing. (N.B.: Do not burst blisters or remove clothing sticking to the burns or scalds).

(b) *Chemical burns* Remove any contaminated clothing which shows no sign of sticking to the skin and flush all affected parts of the body with plenty of clean, cool water ensuring that all the chemical is so diluted as to be rendered harmless. Apply a sterilised dressing to exposed, damaged skin and clean towels to damaged areas where the clothing cannot be removed. (N.B.: Take care when treating the casualty to avoid contamination).

(c) *Foreign bodies in the eye* If the object cannot be removed readily with a clean piece of moist material, irrigate with clean, cool water. People with eye injuries which are more than minimal must be sent to hospital with the eye covered with an eye pad from the container.

(d) *Chemical in the eye* Flush the open eye *at once* with clean, cool water; continue for at least 5 to 10 minutes and, in any case of doubt, even longer. If the contamination is more than minimal, send the casualty to hospital.

(e) *Electric shock* Ensure that the current is switched off. If this is impossible, free the person, using heavy duty insulating gloves (to BS 697/1977) where these are provided for this purpose near the first-aid container, or using something made of rubber, dry cloth or wood or folded newspaper; use the casualty's own clothing if dry. *Be careful* not to touch the casualty's skin before the current is switched off. If breathing is failing or has stopped, start resuscitation and continue until breathing is restored or medical, nursing or ambulance personnel take over.

(f) *Gassing* Move the casualty to fresh air *but make sure that whoever does this is wearing suitable respiratory protection*. If breathing has stopped, start resuscitation and continue until breathing is restored or until medical, nursing or ambulance personnel take over. If the casualty needs to go to hospital make sure a note of the gas involved is sent with him.

General

(a) *Hygiene* When possible, wash your hands before treating wounds, burns or eye injuries. Take care in any event not to contaminate the surfaces of dressings.

(b) *Treatment position* Casualties should be seated or lying down while being treated.

(c) *Record-keeping* An entry must be made in the accident book (for example BI 510 Social Security Act Book) of each case.

(d) *Minor injuries* Casualties with minor injuries of a sort they would attend to themselves if at home may wash their hands and apply a small sterilised dressing from the container.

(e) *First-aid materials* Each article used from the container should be replaced as soon as possible.

THIS LEAFLET IS REPRODUCED BY PERMISSION OF THE
HEALTH & SAFETY EXECUTIVE

Figure 16.1   Official guidance notes issued by the Health and Safety Executive and to be included in all first aid boxes

following injuries it must be reported to the responsible authority by the manager or the person having control of the workplace. In the case of a factory, building site or farm, this is the District Health and Safety Inspector. In the case of an office, shop or restaurant it is the local Environmental Health Department. The first aider may be the first person to deal with the accident that led to the injury, and will be entering it into the *Accident Book*, and may be completing a company accident report. If he or she is aware that an injury falls into the categories listed below the first aider should inform the management.

(a) The death of any person.
(b) Any person suffering from any of the following injuries:
   (i) fracture of the skull, spine or pelvis;
   (ii) fracture of any bone in the arm, wrist, leg or ankle; (not the hand or foot)
   (iii) amputation of a hand, foot, finger, thumb or toe, or any part thereof if the joint or bone are completely severed;
   (iv) the loss of sight in an eye, a penetrating injury or chemical or hot metal burn to an eye;
   (v) an electric shock that has led to loss of consciousness or required immediate medical treatment;
   (vi) loss of consciousness from lack of oxygen;
   (vii) decompression sickness requiring immediate medical treatment, unless suffered during work covered by the Diving Operations at Work Regulations, 1981;
   (viii) acute illness needing treatment, or loss of consciousness from the absorption of any substance by inhalation, ingestion, or through the skin;
   (ix) acute illness from exposure to infected material;
   (x) any other injury that results in the person being admitted immediately to hospital for over 24 hours.

(c) Any person whose injury incapacitates him from work for over 3 days.
(d) The death of any person from an injury within the subsequent year.

Any death, serious injury, or dangerous occurrence must be notified immediately, e.g. by telephone. All reports must be sent in within seven days, on Form F 2508.

Notifiable industrial diseases

It is not part of first aid for the first aider to know the names of all the forty-two industrial diseases and conditions which doctors and management are bound by law to notify to the Health and Safety Inspectorate, local authority or to the Environmental Health Department. But if he or she suspects such a condition management should at once be informed or the occupational health service, if there is one, should be contacted.

The following is the list of notifiable diseases.

(a) Poisoning by:

acrylamide	lead
arsenic	manganese
benzene	mercury
benzene derivatives	methyl bromide
beryllium	oxides of nitrogen
cadmium	phosphorus
carbon disulphide	ethylene oxide
diethylene dioxide	

(b) Skin diseases:

chrome ulcer
folliculitis ⎫
acne ⎬ due to mineral oil, tar,
skin cancer ⎭ pitch or arsenic
radiation skin injury

(c) Lung diseases:

occupational asthma from: isocyanates
platinum salts
hardening agents
rosin flux
proteolytic enzymes
animals or insects used in
laboratories
vegetable dusts

extrinsic alveolitis farmers lung
handling mouldy vegetable
matter or fungi
handling birds
handling bagasse

pneumoconiosis:	from silica, in a wide variety of occupations
byssinosis	from cotton and flax
asbestosis	
lung cancer	from asbestos
mesothelioma	
lung cancer:	from gaseous nickel compounds

(d) Infections:

Leptospirosis:	from rats
Hepatitis:	from infected human blood
Tuberculosis:	from infected humans or animals
Anthrax:	from infected hair or hides or elsewhere

(e) Other conditions:

bone cancer:	
blood dyscrasia:	from ionising radiations
cataract:	from electromagnetic radiation
decompression sickness:	
barotrauma:	from working in conditions of high air pressure
nasal or sinus cancer:	from certain wood dusts, working in the shoe industry, or with gaseous nickel compounds
angiosarcoma of the liver:	from vinyl chloride
cancer of the urinary tract:	from naphthylamine and certain related chemicals
vibration white finger:	from vibrating hand tools

Industrial disablement benefit: role of the DHSS

Under the National Insurance (Industrial Injuries) Act, 1964, a series of regulations has been made recognising that certain diseases can be attributed to the working environment in specified jobs. These diseases are known as *prescribed diseases*. Changes to benefit entitlement were made in the Social Security and Housing Benefits Act, 1982, when short term *industrial injury benefit* was abolished.

Anyone who suffers from any of these prescribed diseases or from the effects of an industrial injury may be able to claim industrial disablement benefit if the condition continues to cause problems. The patient has to make the necessary claim by filling in a form obtained from the local office of the Department of Health and Social Security. Full details are given in free leaflets, also obtainable from the local office:

- NI 2, *Industrial injuries disablement benefit if you have an industrial disease*;
- NI 237, *Occupational asthma*,
- NI 207, *Occupational deafness*,
- NI 3, *Pneumoconiosis or byssinosis*,
- NI 6, *Industrial disablement benefit after an injury at work*

17　First aid in the home

Many industrial first aiders have asked about the proper contents of a first aid box for use in the home or on holiday or in the car. The principles of first aid are exactly the same wherever the patient is injured or taken ill, but the risks are different. The home first aid box should include all that is needed for dealing with minor injuries and illnesses, and the essentials for the emergency first aid treatment of major accidents.

Contents of the home first aid box

Minor wounds
- one tin of assorted individual plaster dressings. These are used surprisingly quickly, so the bigger the tin the better;
- one small (say 4 oz or 100 ml) bottle of cetrimide or hibitane for wound and skin cleaning;
- one plastic gallipot;
- cotton wool in 1 oz (30 g) packs – strip cotton wool dispenser made of cardboard for use in the home can now be obtained from retail chemists. It is specially useful for wound cleaning.

Major wounds
- three large size sterilized wound dressings;
- three medium size sterilized wound dressings.

Accidents
- Three triangular bandages
- Assorted roller bandages
- One crêpe bandage
- One roll of gauze
- One spool of plaster
- Safety pins

- Scissors
- Splinter forceps
- One envelope of cotton-wool applicators, for removing foreign bodies from the eye

For minor ailments, one must have:

- one clinical thermometer;
- the two types of tablets recommended in our industrial first aid boxes – for headaches and sore throats;
- the compound magnesium trisilicate powder, recommended for stomach upsets;
- one tube of tablets for travel sickness;
- one tube of calamine cream or antihistamine for bites;
- one tube of insect repellant.

It is quite unnecessary to include any other dressings, medicines, creams or splints; they are not needed and clutter up the box, making it harder to find what is required. The home first aid box should always have in it a card giving one's own doctor's name and phone number. Some may think it worth while to add also a copy of this book.

Who suffers from accidents in the home?

The enormous majority of those who suffer serious accidents in the home are old people and young children. Falls make up three quarters of all the accidents in old people, with burns and accidental poisoning a long way behind, but still important. In children, burns and scalds are the greatest risks, with accidental poisoning next; for them, however, the danger is greatest outside the home on the roads.

Home accidents and old people

Common disabilities make old people accident prone. Arthritis hampers their movements and also prevents them saving themselves when they fall. Failing eyesight, deafness and loss of sense of smell expose them to danger. Ageing brains and arteries make them careless and forgetful, and they are liable to dizzy spells. Sometimes a sudden illness leads to an accident; for example a stroke may cause an old person to fall down a flight of stairs.

Old people often live in old homes with worn and frayed carpets, little mats ready to slip on the floor, and ill-lit staircases. Their electrical appliances may be old-fashioned and no longer safe. Slippers, worn all day long, may trip them or catch in things or slip when they mount a chair to get at something. Younger relatives can do much to minimise these dangers, though sometimes the old are unwilling to change their ways or their possessions. So the prevention of home accidents in the elderly is often a matter of tactful persuasion.

The treatment of accidents in old people follows the lines set out elsewhere in this book. Fractures are particularly common following falls. Even a slight accident, such as tripping over a mat, can result in a fractured neck of the femur. Burns rapidly lead to shock, and speedy hospital treatment is essential. Gassing accidents and electric shocks may call for artificial respiration. Because they are slow in their movements, old people need more external heat than the young; yet they often have to make do with less. So the shocked old person needs to be kept warm on the way to hospital.

Home accidents and children

A child is a learner, full of curiosity and energy, anxious to explore his or her environment. So those looking after children must anticipate and remove hazards.

- Cots must be safe and baby pillows are to be avoided, because of the risk of suffocation.
- Cat nets are essential for prams left unattended in the garden.
- Stairs should have safety gates.
- Fires should be guarded and the guards fixed to the wall.
- Clothing, especially night clothing, should be of non-inflammable material.
- Gas taps should have safety catches and electrical appliances should be well maintained.
- Tablets, medicines and dangerous liquids (and there are these in every home) should be safely placed on high shelves or in locked cupboards.
- Pots and kettles on stoves should be so placed that their handles cannot be reached.
- Above all, young children should not be left alone in a house.

In dealing with the injured or sick child, and sometimes with its mother, kindly firmness is essential. Do not try to separate mother and child, but reassure both. Children are often more frightened than hurt by an accident, particularly by the sight of blood. Firm pressure to the bleeding point and a general clean-up will often work wonders.

In dealing with the more severe accidents, take note of undue drowsiness or vomiting. These may be serious signs and speedy removal to hospital is essential. Children respond less well than adults to shock, burns, and cold. Severe bleeding must be quickly stopped, burns quickly covered, and removal to hospital organised as quickly as possible. Fractures in children are relatively common, particularly fractures of the clavicle and green-stick fractures of the forearm. Though painful at the time, young bones knit quickly and well.

Mishaps in the prime of life

The most common serious mishaps in adults before old age are coronary thrombosis and accidental or suicidal drug overdose or gassing.

Coronary thrombosis is most common in those who smoke heavily and take little or no exercise. In terms of total numbers affected, it is an even more common result of smoking than lung cancer. Prevention is thus largely a matter for the individual.

The treatment is that of shock. The patient must be kept quiet and still; usually the best position is lying on the back, propped up by three or four pillows. Only a doctor (and sometimes not even he) can diagnose a coronary thrombosis with certainty. The only safe rule is to call the doctor to any patient with signs of shock and pain in the chest or arms.

Gassing accidents in the home are treated precisely as industrial gassing accidents, i.e. removal of the patient from the gas without getting oneself gassed, and if necessary the application of artificial respiration and cardiac massage. Rapid transfer to hospital is essential.

Overdose, usually with sedatives or sleeping tablets, call for immediate hospital treatment. The patient should be placed in the semi-prone position and an ambulance called.

In the prevention of suicidal attempts in depressed people, relatives can play a vital part. If they suspect that suicide is being contemplated, they must inform the patient's doctor at the earliest opportunity, making their fears absolutely explicit.

Index